Table of Contents

CHAPTER ONE

EFFECTIVE CARDIAC PERFORMANCE

Effective management of patients requiring hemodynamic monitoring requires a strong foundation in cardiovascular physiology. This chapter will review the key concepts of cardiovascular performance in the normal adult. Application of this material will be covered in other parts of this book. It is not the intention of this author to cover basic cardiac anatomy and physiology but rather to direct the focus of this chapter to principles and their application to hemodynamic monitoring.

Hemodynamics *is the study of the pressure, flow and movement of blood. It is concerned with the forces generated by the heart and the resulting motion of blood through the cardiovascular system.*

Hemodynamic monitoring *is the use of equipment to evaluate the function and performance of the pumping capacity of the heart and the cardiovascular system.*

Cardiac Muscle—The Basis for Cardiac Function

The cardiac muscle cells have the power to contract in an organized pattern and operate as a pump. The following is a brief review of the physiology of the cardiac muscle.

Cell structure

1. Myocardial cells, or fibers, are long and narrow (**Figure 1.1**). They are the basic unit of the atrial and ventricular myocardium.

2. **Cell types:**

    a. Working myocardial cells generate the contractile force of the heart. They are striated in appearance and are the predominant cells of the atrial and ventricular chambers.

    b. Nodal cells are specialized for pacemaker function. They are found in the sinus node and atrioventricular (AV) node and contract weakly because of few contractile fibers.

    c. Purkinje cells are specialized for rapid conduction of impulses. They are found in the Bundle of His, left and right bundle branches, and throughout the ventricle. They also contract weakly because of few contractile fibers.

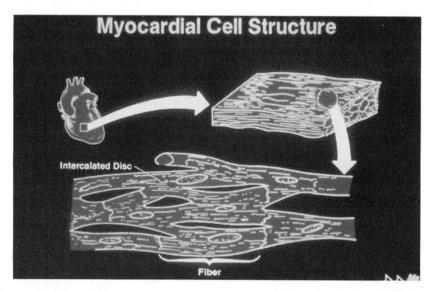

Figure 1.1. Myocardial cells, or fibers, are often branching into a latticework. Each cell is distinct but acts as a coordinated unit. Photo courtesy of Baxter Healthcare Corporation, Edwards Critical-Care Division. Used with permission.

3. A sarcolemma surrounds each cell (**Figure 1.2**). This is a thin elastic sheath of phospholipid and protein that separates the cell contents from the extracellular space. Electrical currents flowing across the sarcolemma initiate contraction.

4. Cells are distinct but are bound end to end to compose cardiac muscle fibers. These cells are connected together at junctions called intercalated discs (**Figure 1.2**). These discs are cell membranes that separate individual cardiac muscle cells from each other.

5. Electrical resistance is minimal through the intercalated discs, and the action potential travels from one cardiac cell to another without significant resistance. Therefore, when one cell becomes excited, the excitation quickly spreads to the others. Because of this property, the heart functions as a syncytium, or fusion, of coordinated cells.

6. Atrial and ventricular syncytium are separate but connected to each other electrically by way of the specialized conduction system of the AV bundle.

7. The myocardial fiber consists of many specialized components. The transverse tubule (T-tubule) system is an extensive network of channels. It carries electrical excitation (calcium ions) to the central portion of the myocardial cells to ensure complete, equal activation (**Figure 1.2**). The T-tubule action potentials cause immediate release of calcium ions from the sarcoplasmic reticulum (SR).

8. The sarcoplasmic reticulum (SR) is an intracellular tubular system with sacs located near the base of each T-tubule. These sacs are sites of calcium storage and release. Calcium is an essential ion which initiates muscle contraction.

9. Mitochondria are sites of the breakdown and resynthesis of the high energy substrate, adenosine triphosphate (ATP). ATP is the energy reservoir which permits cardiac contraction to take place.

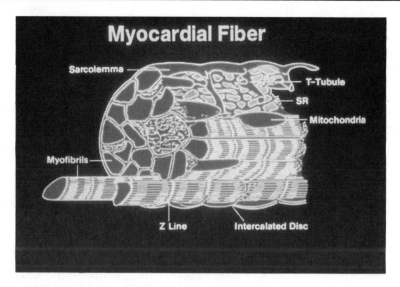

Figure 1.2. The structure of the myocardial fiber allows for the spread of the action potential into the interior of the muscle fiber along the T-tubule, with a release of calcium from the sarcoplasmic reticulum. Photo courtesy of Baxter Healthcare Corporation, Edwards Critical-Care Division. Used with permission.

Myocardial Contraction

Refer to **Figure 1.3** for the following review of myocardial contraction.

1. The sarcomere is the basic functional and structural unit of the myofibril, the contractile element of the muscle fiber. It contains thin and thick filaments which overlap each other in varying amounts depending upon whether the cells are in a state of relaxation or contraction. The filaments are composed of contractile proteins, actin and myosin.

2. At the end of each sarcomere are dark stained Z bands which are attached to the thin filaments. The thin filament is mainly composed of actin. The Z bands indicate the end of one sarcomere and the beginning of the next.

3. The thick filament comprises the center of the sarcomere and consists primarily of myosin.

4. Electrical stimulation of the cardiac cell via the T-tubules triggers the release of calcium from the SR. At that time extra quantities of calcium diffuse from the T-tubules into the myocardial fiber. Circulating calcium binds with proteins, troponin and tropomyosin allowing actin and myosin to interact and contraction to take place. The crossbridges link the thick and thin filaments by moving the thin filament towards the center of the sarcomere. It is the large quantity of calcium that diffuses from the T-tubules which differentiates cardiac from skeletal muscles. This amount of calcium enables the cardiac muscle to maintain a longer contraction than the skeletal muscle.

5. Tropomyosin and troponin, located on the thin filaments, inhibit the interaction of myosin and actin, and the muscle relaxes.

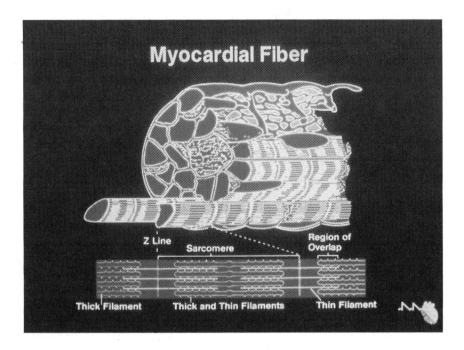

Figure 1.3. The light and dark appearance of the sarcomere is the result of the two proteins, actin and myosin. With contraction, the Z lines move closer together. Photo courtesy of Baxter Healthcare Corporation, Edwards Critical-Care Division. Used with permission.

Cardiac Nerves

The heart has an extensive network of nerve fibers from the sympathetic and parasympathetic nervous systems.

1. Cholinergic fibers arise from the vagus nerve and adrenergic fibers arise from the thoracolumbar sympathetic system to innervate the heart.

2. The atria are innervated by both systems which play an important role in impulse formation, impulse conduction, and force of contraction.

3. The ventricles are mainly innervated by the sympathetic nerve fibers which play a role in conduction and force of contractility.

Cardiac Cycle

The cardiac cycle is primarily a mechanical event. However, electrical activity always precedes mechanical activity. For a discussion of electrical activity, refer to the references at the end of this chapter.

The function of the heart is basically twofold—to receive blood and to distribute blood. This is represented by the systolic and diastolic phases of the cardiac cycle. The period from the end of one heart contraction to the end of the next is the cardiac cycle (**Figure 1.4**).

Systole

This is the period of the cycle when the ventricles are contracting. It can be separated into two phases: isometric (isovolumetric) contraction and ejection phase (**Figure 1.4**).

1. Isometric (isovolumetric) contraction means that there is an increased tension (pressure) in the muscle but no change in intraventricular volume nor shortening of the muscle fibers. Isometric contraction phase marks the onset of ventricular systole and contraction. The ventricular pressure rises rapidly causing the atrioventricular (AV) valves to close. This produces the first heart sound, S_1 (**lub**-dub), and coincides with the peak of the R wave. The aortic and pulmonary valves have not yet opened. The ventricles need to develop sufficient pressure to push open the aortic and pulmonic valves against the pressures in the aorta and pulmonary artery. During this time contraction occurs, but no emptying takes place. When ventricular pressure exceeds aortic and pulmonary artery pressures, the ejection phase begins.

2. Ejection phase is marked by the opening of the aortic and pulmonic valves, muscle shortening, and the rapid ejection of blood. The first quarter of this phase is rapid ejection of 60% of the blood to be ejected from the ventricle. The remaining 40% is ejected in the next two quarters. During the last quarter of this phase, little blood is ejected into the aorta. Both aortic and ventricular pressure decline, and when the ventricular pressure becomes lower than the aortic pressure, the aortic and pulmonic valves close. The amount of blood that is left in the ventricle at the end of systole is called the end-systolic volume or residual. This amount is normally about 50-60 milliliters (ml) and varies with the contractile state of the heart.

Diastole

This is the period of the cycle when the ventricles are relaxing. It can be divided into the following four phases (**Figure 1.4**):

1. Isometric (isovolumetric) relaxation is marked by the closure of the aortic and pulmonic valves while the AV valves have not yet opened. This produces the second heart sound, S_2 (lub-**dub**). The closure of the aortic valve produces the dicrotic notch, noted on the arterial wave form. There is a rapid decline in ventricular pressure but no change in volume as both sets of valves are closed. When the ventricular pressure is below the atrial pressure, the AV valves open.

2. Rapid ventricular filling occurs when the AV valves have opened, and the blood flows rapidly from the atria to the ventricles.

3. Slow ventricular filling is marked by slow movement of blood from the atria to the ventricles, and contributes only a small additional volume of blood to the ventricles.

4. Atrial systole is marked by contraction of the atria and contributes an additional 30% blood supply to the ventricles (atrial kick). This is the end of ventricular filling and ventricular diastole. The volume of blood in the ventricles (usually 120-130 ml) at this time is called left ventricular end-diastolic volume (LVEDV) and is measured as left ventricular end-diastolic pressure (LVEDP).

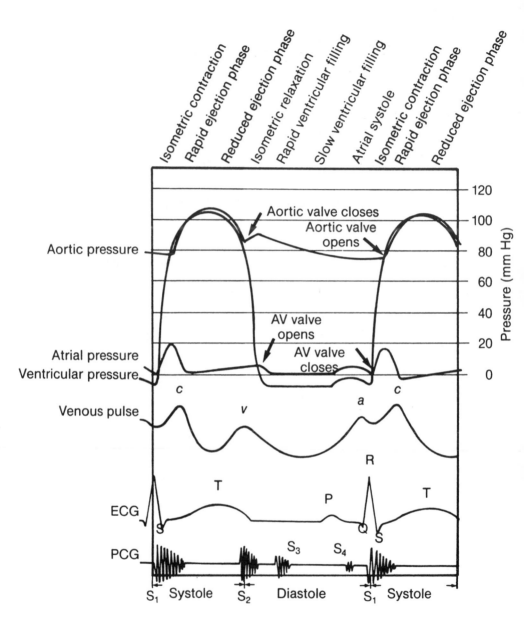

Figure 1.4. Events of the cardiac cycle. Shows ventricular pressures in systole and diastole, ECG, heart sounds (phonocardiogram), and venous pressures. Mary Canobbio, *Cardiovascular Disorders: Clinical Nursing Series,* Saint Louis: Mosby-Year Book,1990. Used with permission of the publisher.

Cardiac Output

The heart is a muscular pump and propels the blood through the circulatory system via the vascular network. The performance of the pump is described in terms of cardiac output.

Cardiac output (CO) is the amount of blood pumped by the left ventricle into the aorta in one minute. It is measured in liters per minute. Cardiac output varies with body size. Generally the normal CO is 4-8 Liters/minute (**Figure 1.5**).

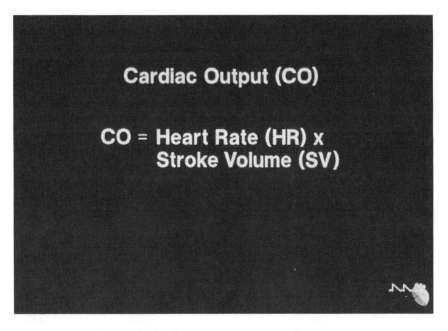

Figure 1.5. A mathematical representation of cardiac output. Photo courtesy of Baxter Healthcare Corporation, Edwards Critical-Care Division. Used with permission.

Cardiac Index (CI) is a number obtained by dividing cardiac output by the body surface area. This takes into consideration the individual differences in height and weight. Normal values are 2.5-4.0 Liters/minute/m^2. See appendix 2 for formulas.

Stroke volume (SV) is the amount of blood pumped by the left ventricle into the aorta with each contraction. It is measured in milliliters per contraction or beat. Normal values are 60-100 milliliters/beat. Stroke volume can also be indexed to body surface area. Normal values are 40-50 ml/m^2. See appendix 2 for formulas.

Ejection fraction is the ratio of the volume of blood that is ejected from the left ventricle with each beat (SV) to the volume of blood in the left ventricle at the end of diastole (LVEDV). The normal ejection fraction in the adult is about 65% plus or minus 8. Ejection fraction can be calculated by the following equation: EF = $^{SV}/_{LVEDV}$. The ejection fraction is an indication of the systolic performance of the left ventricle as a pump.

Cardiac reserve is the ability of the heart to increase its output in situations where oxygen requirements are increased. In the healthy adult, normal cardiac output can be increased up to 5 times the resting needs. In contrast, in a diseased heart, the resting needs may already be utilizing the cardiac reserve, and the person has limited ability to increase the cardiac output.

Factors Affecting Cardiac Output

Figure 1.5 shows that the calculation of cardiac output equals heart rate times stroke volume. Stroke volume is dependent upon preload, afterload, and contractility which operate simultaneously to determine effective cardiac performance. **Figure 1.6** represents the four major determinants of cardiac output. They are:
- Preload
- Afterload
- Contractility
- Heart rate

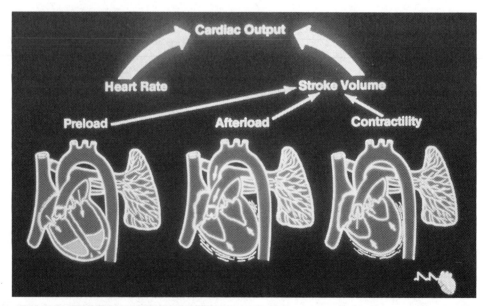

Figure 1.6. Factors affecting cardiac output. Photo courtesy of Baxter Healthcare Corporation, Edwards Critical-Care Division. Used with permission.

Preload

This is the amount of blood that is present in the ventricles at the end of diastole. In the resting phase of diastole, the heart muscle is stretched and a resting tension or resting pressure develops. This is the measurement of preload. Simultaneously, during systole, this blood is pumped out of the pulmonary artery to the lungs and out of the aortic valve to the aorta. **Figure 1.7** represents the various factors which affect preload. They are:

1. Venous return—the amount of blood that flows into the heart each minute. The actual amount is dependent upon:

    a. The local blood flow through all the individual tissues of the body.

    b. The rate of venous return from the peripheral vessels back to the heart. This is directly related to the average effective pressure of the blood in the peripheral circulation. That is to say, the circulatory system must have enough volume to maintain a peripheral pressure that will push the blood back to the right ventricle (see peripheral circulatory system). Pressures in the right atrium must remain normally low or the resistance to blood flow would cause back pressure on the systemic circulation and decrease venous return. Under normal circumstances, the amount of blood that returns to the right side of the heart presents itself in the left ventricle during diastolic filling, and this blood is pumped into the systemic circulation around the circuit again.

2. End-systolic volume—the amount of blood that remains in the heart after systole.

3. Atrial systole—may contribute an additional 30% blood supply to the ventricles (atrial kick).

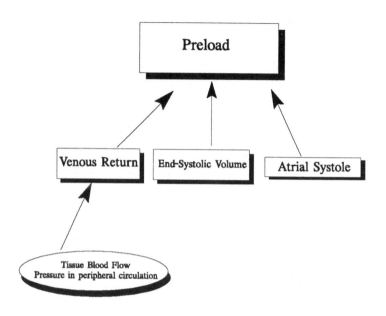

Figure 1.7. Factors affecting preload.

Myocardial stretch is the degree to which the muscle fibers are stretched during diastole. This stretch is a reflection of preload and ventricular compliance. Two physiologists, Frank and Starling, stated that the heart muscle has the intrinsic ability to adapt itself to changing amounts of blood (**Figure 1.8**). To a point, the more the heart is filled during diastole, the larger the volume of blood pumped into the aorta (SV). Within physiological limits, the heart muscle can stretch and pump small or large quantities of blood as long as the quantity is not beyond the heart's ability. The stretched muscle responds with a greatly increased force of contraction. The stretch of the sarcomere to 2.2 microns produces the maximal contractile force. In the normal heart, at this optimal stretch, the ventricular end-diastolic volume (preload) is approximately 12 mm Hg. As **Figure 1.8** indicates, an over or under stretch of the muscle will produce a less than maximal stroke volume and cardiac output. The heart behaves in this predictable manner as long as the afterload and contractility remain constant. In the normal heart, the ventricle can accommodate large diastolic volumes with only a small increase in diastolic resting tension.

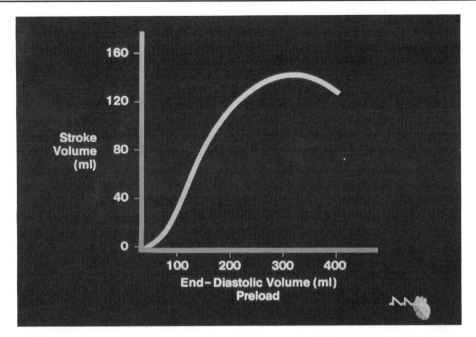

Figure 1.8. A graphic representation of the Frank-Starling Law. The end-diastolic volume is also the end-diastolic pressure. As the muscle is stretched beyond a certain point, the stroke volume and cardiac output decreases. Photo courtesy of Baxter Healthcare Corporation, Edwards Critical-Care Division. Used with permission.

Afterload

This is the force the heart muscle must generate to eject the blood from the left ventricle into the peripheral circulation. In other words, it is the systemic resistance to flow. Afterload (**Figure 1.9**) is dependent upon impedence to left ventricular ejection with such situations as:

1. Increased or decreased systemic vascular resistance

2. Outflow obstructions, such as aortic valve stenosis. Left ventricular pressure must exceed aortic pressure in order for the aortic valve to open. A stenotic valve creates a resistance that the left ventricle must overcome in order to open the aortic valve.

3. Ventricular dilatation: With increased outflow impedence, there is a decrease in stroke volume and cardiac output. When impedence is lowered, stroke volume increases. The systemic vascular resistance (SVR) is an indicator of the left ventricular afterload. This is a calculated number (see the appendix) using the mean arterial pressure, central venous pressure and the cardiac output. In the absence of these numbers, the mean arterial pressure (see the appendix) can be used as an approximation of the SVR.

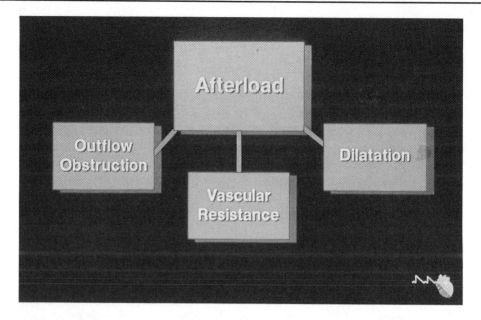

Figure 1.9. Factors affecting afterload. Photo courtesy of Baxter Healthcare Corporation, Edwards Critical-Care Division. Used with permission.

Contractility

Contractility is an inherent property of the heart muscle to contract. (See muscle contraction for further discussion). Cardiac muscle has a longer sustained depolarization period than other types of muscles. The depolarization period is much longer at slow heart rates than at rapid ones.

When the cardiac muscle is exposed to such factors as pharmacological influences, oxygen imbalance, electrolyte disturbances, sympathetic or parasympathetic stimulation, and hormonal influences, the contractile force will be altered. Contractility is not the same as cardiac performance **(Figure 1.10)**. While it is certainly one factor in determining the effectiveness of cardiac performance, other previously described factors need to be taken into account.

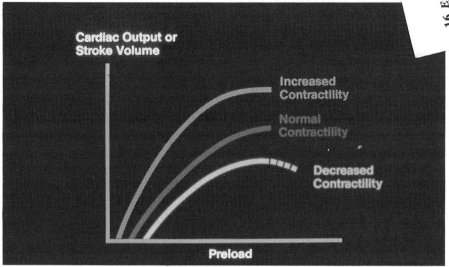

Figure 1.10. Contractility is a factor affecting cardiac output. For a given preload, a decrease in contractility will move the curve to the right and produce a decreased stroke volume and cardiac output. An increase in contractility will produce an increased stroke volume and cardiac output. Photo courtesy of Baxter Healthcare Corporation, Edwards Critical-Care Division. Used with permission.

Heart Rate

Heart rate (HR) is the number of contractions per minute. The heart muscle is stimulated, via the electrical conduction pathways, to produce a mechanical contraction which is either auscultated or palpated. A change in the heart rate and rhythm can quickly change cardiac output. An increase in the force of contraction with an increase in heart rate is called the "staircase phenomenon." This will occur with a sinus mechanism up to the rate of about 150 at which time the force of contraction will plateau. Even though the diastolic filling time is decreased with rapid heart rates, this increase in force of contraction provides compensation up to a point. This benefit is not seen with ectopic tachycardias. In rates that are bradycardiac (below 60) or tachycardiac (above 100), the cardiac output may fall.

Regulation of Heart Rate

The heart rate is principally controlled by the **autonomic nervous system**.

1. Direct stimulation of the sinoatrial node by the sympathetic nervous system increases heart rate and facilitates increased AV conduction, while stimulation of the parasympathetic nervous system decreases heart rate and slows AV conduction. In the healthy resting adult, the parasympathetic tone predominates. Sympathetic stimulation not only increases heart rate but also increases contractility. Heart rate also increases in response to catecholamines, epinephrine and norepinephrine, released directly into the circulating blood by the adrenal medulla. In this way, there are two systems for stimulating the heart.

2. Emotional states, such as anxiety, excitement, or rage, can initiate changes in heart rates by direct stimulation of the sympathetic nervous system.

3. **Baroreceptors** play an important role in the regulation of heart rate as a result of their significant role in the short-term control of arterial blood pressure. These baroreceptors are located in the aortic arch and carotid sinuses. Changes in heart rate occur in response to activity of the two branches of the autonomic nervous system. For example, when the patient becomes hypotensive, the baroreceptors sense this information and send impulses:

   a. To the medulla for vasoconstriction.

   b. To the vagus nerve for inhibition to allow an increased heart rate and strength of contraction. Changes in heart rate take place within 1-2 seconds.

4. **Atrial receptors** increase heart rate in response to stretch in the atria and are located in the right atrium at the junction of the venae cavae and in the left atrium at the junction of the pulmonary veins. The increased volume in the atria stretches the sinoatrial node, the pacemaker of the heart. Heart rate can increase as much as 75%.

   Another control of heart rate is due to the effect of the Bainbridge reflex. The atrial stretch receptors send impulses to the vasomotor center which transmits signals back via the sympathetic and vagal nerves to increase the rate and strength of contraction. The magnitude of the response depends upon the existing heart rate. A very slow rate will increase heart rate; a very fast rate will slow the heart rate. However, under normal circumstances, increased filling elicits tachycardia.

5. **Chemoreceptors** are also located near the aortic arch and carotid sinuses. They are indirectly responsible for changes in heart rate. This is best illustrated by the following example. When the carotid chemoreceptors are

stimulated by a low carbon dioxide, the ventilatory depth and rate increases. It is the change in pulmonary ventilation that creates the change in the heart rate.

Myocardial Work, Oxygen Consumption, Oxygen Delivery

Myocardial Work

As with other muscles, the heart requires a constant energy source for muscle contraction and ion transport. At any one time the energy source is sufficient to produce only a few minutes of activity. The metabolism of free fatty acids provides the major energy source for myocardial activity. Under anaerobic or ischemic conditions, cardiac metabolism utilizes anaerobic glycolysis for energy. This mechanism supplies very little energy and at the same time produces large amounts of lactic acid. The energy requirements depend upon the amount and type of work the heart is doing.

Work can be defined as the ejection of a volume of blood under pressure and as the product of pressure times stroke volume ($P \times SV$). In other words, it is the amount of work performed in moving blood from the right ventricle into the pulmonary artery and from the left ventricle into the aorta. The stroke volume of both ventricles is the same, but since the aortic pressure is higher than the pulmonic pressure, the pressure volume work of the left ventricle is approximately seven times that of the right ventricle.

Any changes in the components of pressure or stroke volume will change the amount of work the heart muscle must accomplish. (See the previous discussion of stroke volume, preload, and afterload.) **Figure 1.11** demonstrates how afterload is inversely related to stroke volume and directly related to the oxygen consumption (MVO_2) by cardiac tissues.

Myocardial Oxygen Supply

Blood flow through the coronary system is regulated by the nutritional needs of the cardiac muscle. The greater the work, the greater the need for oxygen, and the greater the oxygen consumption. Under normal conditions, the heart extracts between 65-80% of the oxygen delivered to it. When oxygen demands are increased such as during exercise, little extra oxygen can be extracted! The additional oxygen can be supplied only by increasing coronary blood flow. If the blood flow fails to increase to meet demands, the strength of the muscle diminishes, often causing acute heart failure.

Myocardial Oxygen Consumption (MVO₂)

The rate of blood flow is determined by oxygen demand and consumption. The major determinants of myocardial oxygen consumption are:

1. Ventricular wall tension or pressure in the walls of the ventricles. Tension is a function of the internal pressure and radius of the ventricular cavity and thickness of the ventricular wall. Therefore, any change in preload or afterload may affect tension.

2. Velocity of shortening of myocardial fibers, or rate of development of tension

3. Degree of shortening of myocardial fibers

4. Increased metabolic activity from epinephrine, norepinephrine, increased temperature of the heart, and/or inotropic agents. Increases in heart rate also increase myocardial oxygen consumption.

The balance between the work that is done by the myocardium and the energy used to produced this work is cardiac efficiency. Generally, efficiency improves with volume loading (Frank-Starling's Law) and diminishes with increased afterload (**Figure 1.10 and 1.11**).

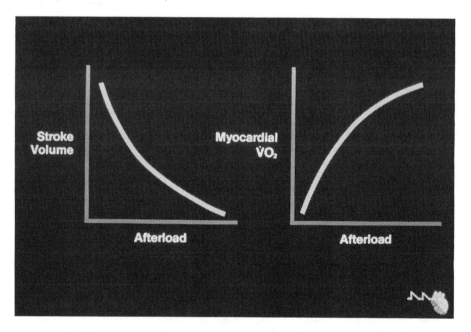

Figure 1.11. The greater the afterload, the less the stroke volume. The greater the afterload, the greater the myocardial oxygen consumption (VO₂). Photo courtesy of Baxter Healthcare Corporation, Edwards Critical-Care Division. Used with permission.

Coronary Blood Flow

The coronary blood supply is delivered through the right coronary artery, the left anterior descending artery, the left circumflex artery and the branches of each of these arteries. The epicardial or surface vessels are large and the intramuscular arteries are smaller. The latter penetrate the muscle on their way down to the endocardium. During systolic contraction, the heart muscle squeezes towards the center of the ventricle and blood flow through the smaller intramuscular arteries of the coronary system is interrupted and falls to near zero.

The pressure during systole is greatest near the endocardial surface and becomes progressively less towards the epicardial surface. During diastole, the cardiac muscle relaxes and blood flows rapidly into the subendocardial layer. Blood flow through the right ventricle undergoes similar, but milder, changes through systole and diastole because the force of contraction of the right ventricle is less than that of the left ventricle. The driving force for perfusion of the coronary arteries is the pressure at the root of the aorta during diastole.

Autoregulation tends to keep coronary perfusion stable regardless of changes in coronary perfusion pressure within limits of about 60 to 180 mm Hg. However, when coronary perfusion pressure falls below approximately 60 mm Hg, autoregulation is lost. At approximately 40 mm Hg, the coronary arteries collapse, and flow stops. It is essential to maintain a perfusion pressure of 60 to 80 mm Hg to prevent collapse of the coronary arteries.

Hemodynamics of the Peripheral Circulatory System

A functional relationship exists between the central venous pressure and cardiac output. This relationship depends upon:
- Peripheral resistance
- Arterial capacitance
- Venous capacitance

The following reviews the interaction of these factors.

Key Concepts of Flow, Pressure and Resistance

1. An important factor in determining the rate of blood flow through a vessel is the diameter of the blood vessel. Changes in the diameter of the vessel can cause enormous changes in the amount of blood that is propelled. For instance, a change in the diameter of a vessel from 2 ml to 4 ml can increase blood flow from 16 ml/minute to 256 ml/minute.

2. Overall blood flow is actually the cardiac output because it is the amount of blood pumped by the heart in a unit of time. Venous return usually equals cardiac output over a period of time.

3. Blood flow is laminar flow. This means that within the blood vessel, blood lies in a series of individual layers, each of which is moving at a different velocity. The blood near the vessel wall moves slowly, the next layer of blood moves a little more quickly, but the central layers move rapidly.

4. Turbulent flow implies that blood is flowing in all directions in the vessel and is continually mixing within the vessel. This occurs when blood passes by an obstruction or over a rough surface. There is always some turbulent flow in the proximal portions of the aorta and pulmonary artery and during rapid ejection phase of systole. Turbulent flow can be detected by murmurs. Intravascular thrombosis is more likely to occur with turbulent than laminar flow.

5. Pressure is also another determinant of the rate of flow (**Figure 1.12**). The pressure difference between two ends of a vessel determines the rate of flow. Blood flows from an area of high pressure to an area of low pressure. The pressure difference is responsible for propelling blood through a vessel.

6. The principal factor in resistance to blood flow within the circulatory system is the caliber of the vessel. The resistance to flow is inversely related to the diameter of the vessel. The greater the diameter of the vessel, the less the resistance to flow. The greatest resistance to flow is in the arterioles. Constriction of the smooth muscle cells in the vessel walls change the radius of the vessel.

7. Resistance to flow is related to the blood viscosity. The greater the viscosity of blood, the greater the resistance. Hematocrit and albumin are indicators of resistance to blood flow based on viscosity.

When calculating total systemic vascular resistance during hemodynamic monitoring, the term systemic vascular resistance is used instead of total peripheral resistance. Refer to the appendix for the formula.

The resistance to flow increases from the aorta to the arterioles to the capillaries. The velocity of the blood flow is inversely proportional to its cross sectional area (**Figure 1.12**). The cross-sectional area of the capillary bed is large even though the cross-sectional area of each capillary is small. As a result, blood flows through the capillaries very slowly. Pressure falls progressively from the aorta through the systemic circulation to approximately 0 mm Hg by the time it reaches the right atrium. As the blood returns to the right heart, the velocity of blood flow increases.

Capacitance

The greatest resistance to flow is in the arterioles. The arteries are more muscular than veins and are not distensible. Venous capacitance is about twenty times as great as arterial capacitance (**Figure 1.12**). The veins are storage areas for blood. The volume of blood in the arterial system is only about 11% whereas 67% of blood volume is in the venous system.

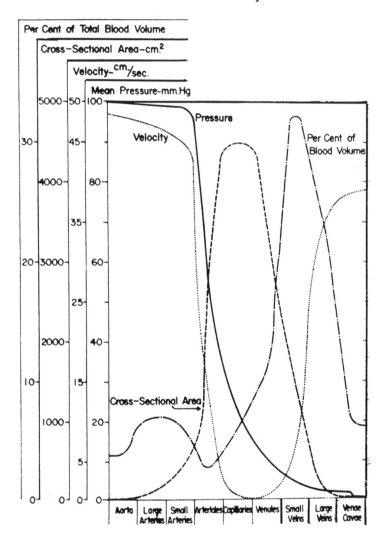

Figure 1.12. Pressure, velocity of flow, cross-sectional area, and capacity of the blood vessels of the systemic circulation.

The important features are the inverse relationship between the velocity and cross-sectional area, the major pressure drop across the arterioles, the maximal cross-sectional area and minimal flow rate in the capillaries, and the large capacity of the venous system. The small, but abrupt, drop in pressure in the venae cavae indicates the point of entrance of these vessels into the thoracic cavity and reflects the effect of the negative intrathoracic pressure. To permit schematic representation of velocity and cross-sectional area on a single linear scale, only approximations are possible at the lower values. Robert Berne and Matthew Levy, *Cardiovascular Physiology,* (6th edition) Saint Louis: Mosby-Year Book, 1992. Used with permission of the publisher.

Control of Peripheral Blood Flow and Pressure

The peripheral circulation is controlled centrally by the nervous system and locally by the tissue's need for blood flow. Autoregulation is the control of local blood flow through the tissue in response to its needs for nutrients and oxygen, independent of the nervous system. Factors which control local blood flow are:

- Rate of tissue metabolism
- Oxygen, carbon dioxide levels
- Specific function of the tissue/organ

Central Control of Blood Flow

1. Regions in the pons and medulla, called the vasomotor center, control sympathetic activity. The hypothalamus and the cerebral cortex can exert inhibitory or excitatory effects on the vasomotor centers. This area picks up signals from all over the body and transmits them from this area downwards through the spinal cord to all peripheral vessels. Sympathetic nerves from the vasomotor center innervate arteries, arterioles, venules and veins. Stimulation causes the arteries and arterioles to increase their resistance, change the rate of flow through them, and produce blood pressure changes.

2. "Stressors" can cause direct sympathetic nerve stimulation. Impulses are transmitted downward through the spinal cord to the smooth muscles of the peripheral vessels. Norepinephrine is the substance that is secreted at the end of the sympathetic nerve endings. It acts directly upon the smooth muscles of the vessel to cause vasoconstriction.

3. In addition, the adrenal medulla secretes large amounts of counter-regulatory hormones, norepinephrine and epinephrine, into the circulating blood which in response to sympathetic impulses, cause vasoconstriction.

4. Baroreceptors and chemoreceptors are rapid-acting pressure control mechanisms. Baroreceptors respond to the stretch of the walls of the major arteries (e.g. carotids and aortic arch) in the chest and neck. The stretch excites the baroreceptors and sends signals back to the vasomotor center, which in turn transmits signals back to the vessels to relax and dilate. Chemoreceptors are sensitive to decreases in levels of oxygen and increases in carbon dioxide due to low blood flow. Signals are transmitted to the vasomotor center to "excite" this area and elevate blood pressure back to normal.

5. Increases in blood volume in the central veins and in the atria excite stretch receptors. In response, the vasomotor center, kidneys, and the hypothalamus control the amount of blood volume back to normal.

6. Renin is secreted by the kidney in response to a decrease in arterial pressure. This enzyme acts on plasma protein to form angiotensin I. Within the lung, angiotensin I is converted to angiotensin II. Angiotensin II is a potent vasoconstrictor and thereby elevates arterial pressure. For long-term pressure management, angiotensin II is a catalyst for the production and release of aldosterone from the adrenal cortex. Aldosterone then stimulates sodium reabsorption by the renal tubules and the water that accompanies the sodium. This produces an increase in blood pressure.

7. Vasopressin, the antidiuretic hormone, is a potent vasoconstricting agent. It is formed in the hypothalamus but is secreted by the posterior pituitary gland. It also controls volume by controlling water reabsorption in the renal tubules.

8. Endothelins (signalling peptides) secreted by the endothelium of vessel walls act as highly potent localized vasoconstrictors and can be stimulated by epinephrine and angiotensin II or inhibited by atrial natriuretic peptide.

9. Other vasodilator substances such as bradykinin, serotonin, histamine, and prostaglandins play a role in pressure regulation.

10. Increases in potassium, magnesium, sodium, pH, and CO_2 can dilate local blood vessels, although their role in regulation of flow is not determined.

Summary

The principles covered in this chapter are the key concepts of cardiovascular performance in the normal adult. These principles must be understood and mastered. They are the foundation on which to build when assessing the more complicated, critical care patient who will require hemodynamic monitoring.

Selected References

Berne, Robert M., Levy, and Matthew N. *Cardiovascular Physiology.* (6th edition) Saint Louis: The C.V. Mosby Company, 1992.

Canobbio, Mary M. *Cardiovascular Disorders.* Clinical Nursing Series. Saint Louis: The C.V. Mosby Company, 1990.

Cheitlin, M., Sokolow, Maurice, and McIlroy, Malcolm. *Clinical Cardiology.* (6th edition) Connecticut: Appelton & Lange, 1993.

Daily, Elaine, and Schroeder, John. *Techniques in Bedside Hemodynamic Monitoring.* (5th edition) Saint Louis: The C.V. Mosby Company, 1994.

Guyton, Arthur C. *Textbook of Medical Physiology.* (8th edition) Philadelphia: W.B. Saunders Company, 1990.

Katz, Arnold. *Physiology of the Heart.* (2nd edition) New York: Raven Press, 1992.

Kinney, M., Packa, D., and Dunbar, S., *AACN'S Clinical Reference for Critical Care Nursing.* (3rd edition) Saint Louis: C.V. Mosby Company, 1993.

Little, Robert, and Little, William. *Physiology of the Heart and Circulation.* (4th edition) Chicago: Year Book Medical Publishers, Inc., 1989.

Thelan, L., Davie, J., Urden, L., and Lough, M. *Critical Care Nursing, Diagnosis and Management.* (2nd edition), 1994.

CHAPTER TWO

PRINCIPLES OF NON-INVASIVE CARDIOVASCULAR ASSESSMENT

Critical care nurses must master the skills and techniques of interview, inspection, palpation, percussion, and auscultation to complete a comprehensive assessment of the cardiovascular system. Examination and evaluation of the patient's general appearance, vital signs, arterial pressures, venous pressures and the heart will be reviewed in this chapter. Data obtained through histories and physical examination should be compiled with invasive, hemodynamic monitoring measurements to identify problems and to plan and provide optimum care for critically ill patients.

Comprehensive Cardiovascular History

Through interviewing the patient, a thorough history should be obtained that will help to identify cardiac problems. In the critical care setting, it is often difficult to obtain a thorough history from the patient. Very often there is a need to rely on information given the nurse by family members or by other members of the health care team. Ideally, the history should include the patient's chief complaint, history of present illness, past medical history, review of systems, social history, and any pertinent family history.

1. **Chief complaint** (CC)—Why is the patient seeking medical care? It is important to use "patient's own words" whenever possible.

2. **History of present illness** (HPI)—Determine:
   - Date and time of onset
   - Description of complaint
   - Mode of onset, course, duration
   - Associated signs and symptoms:
     - Pain—character, location, radiation, quality, duration, factors that aggravate or produce, and factors that alleviate. Rate pain on a scale of 1-10 (1 as no pain and 10 as most severe pain ever experienced).
     - Fatigue—with or without activity
     - Edema—location, degree, AM or PM occurrence
     - Syncope—with or without dizziness, and time of occurrence
     - Dyspnea, orthopnea, paroxysmal nocturnal dyspnea, dyspnea on exertion
     - Palpitations
     - Hemoptysis
     - Cyanosis (circumoral, extremities)
     - Intermittent claudication
     - Clubbing of fingernails

3. **Past medical history**—This includes all previous illnesses, injuries, hospitalizations, surgical procedures, and **allergies**. Information regarding current medication use should be obtained. Include all prescription and over-the-counter (OTC) medications and note name, dosage, route, frequency, and the patient's reason for taking them.

4. **Social history**—obtain information about your patient's life-style patterns and personal habits. Include:
   - Educational background

- Present and past work experiences
- Exercise and recreational activities
- Use of alcohol/tobacco/recreational drugs/caffeine. Note pack/year history for smokers (# cigarettes/day for how many years)
- Dietary habits
- Potential stressors
- Relationships with significant others

5. **Family history**—includes the state of health or cause of death of immediate family members. The hereditary/familial diseases pertaining to the cardiovascular system which should be noted include:

- Diabetes mellitus
- Hypertension
- Cardiovascular disease (MI, CAD, CHF)
- Gout
- Obesity
- Hyperlipidemia
- Renal disease
- Peripheral vascular disease (CVA or TIA's)

Cardiovascular Physical Examination

A systematic physical examination should be done to investigate any abnormalities the patient's history or symptoms suggest. The techniques of inspection, palpation, percussion, and auscultation should be used to perform the physical exam. Evaluation of the patient's general appearance, vital signs, arterial pulses, venous jugular system, and examination of the heart should be conducted. In the acutely ill patient, physical examination is usually performed with vital signs. Any changes in the assessment should be recorded in the patient's record and reported to the physician/other members of the health care team.

Inspection involves visual observation or the use of the "eyes" to capture normal and abnormal findings ("looking with a purpose").

Palpation utilizes the sense of touch to examine body tissues and organs.

Percussion involves tapping body surfaces to elicit sounds. These sounds help to determine the position, size and density of underlying structures, as well as air or fluid levels.

Auscultation involves using the ear to recognize respiratory, cardiac and vascular sounds. A stethoscope with a bell and diaphragm will be most useful in determining the frequency, intensity, quality and duration of each sound heard.

General Appearance

Begin with an overview of patient's physical appearance.

1. Observe for signs of breathing or circulation difficulties. i.e. increased effort or work of breathing, capillary refill.

2. Estimate the patient's age and compare with chronological age.

3. Determine state of nourishment.

4. Assess level of consciousness—note any signs of restlessness, agitation, or irritability. An alteration in the patient's consciousness level can be the result of decreased oxygen supply to the brain. This can occur with decreased cardiac output.

5. Evaluate skin and mucous membranes.

6. Observe for central or peripheral cyanosis:
   - **Central cyanosis** is due to poor oxygenation of arterial blood in the lungs. It refers to bluish discoloration of the tongue, mucous membranes of the mouth, and conjunctiva.
   - **Peripheral cyanosis** occurs when the peripheral tissues extract more oxygen, resulting in a decrease in the amount of hemoglobin in the venous blood. The nailbeds, earlobes, tip of nose, lips, hands and feet become bluish in color.

7. Observe for pallor which is caused by decreased blood flow in the periphery.

8. Observe for clubbing which may be a sign of chronic oxygen deficiency and may be associated with certain cardiac and pulmonary diseases. The angle between the fingernail and nail base is altered, and the nail base may feel spongy or springlike.

9. Inspect the skin for petechiae, and xanthomas (cholesterol-filled nodules on the eyelids and ears).

10. Determine if edema is present. Edema accompanies right-sided heart failure and is usually found in dependent areas of the body including the hands, feet and sacral area.

Vital Signs

1. Temperature

2. Pulse rate—apical and radial:
   - Palpate both radial pulses simultaneously and compare rate, rhythm, and character.

3. Respiratory rate, rhythm and quality

4. Blood pressure:

   a. Appropriate sized cuff should be utilized.

   b. Blood pressure in both arms should be recorded in supine, sitting, and standing positions. A fall in blood pressure of greater than 20 mm Hg when the patient stands indicates excessive orthostatic changes. This may be indicative of blood volume deficits but also may be the result of bleeding, excessive diuretics, or anti-hypertensive drugs.

   - **Pulse pressure,** the difference between systolic and diastolic pressure, is usually 40 mm Hg. It is altered by any factors which influence stroke volume or arterial resistance.

   - **Decreased pulse pressure** (less than 30 mm Hg) may be related to factors which increase diastolic pressure, decrease systolic pressure, or both:
     - It is often an early clinical indication of impending cardiogenic shock, when severe peripheral vasoconstriction and decreased cardiac output are present.

     - It may also be seen when there is a decreased stroke volume, as in congestive heart failure, hypovolemia, and tachycardia.

     - Mechanical causes such as aortic valve stenosis, mitral valve obstructions, or mitral insufficiency may also produce a decreased pulse pressure.

   - **Increased pulse pressure** (greater than 50 mm Hg) is seen when the systolic pressure increases, the diastolic pressure decreases, or both:
     - May be seen with arteriosclerosis and aging when there is a decreased distensibility of the aorta, arteries and arterioles.

     - May also occur with aortic insufficiency.

     - Can be present with arrhythmias such as sinus bradycardia or complete heart block.

     - Silent gaps between systolic and diastolic pressures indicate an auscultatory gap. This may be present in hypertensive patients.

Arterial Pulses

1. Palpation of arterial pulses gives information about systemic circulation and cardiac function.

2. Pulses are produced as a result of the ejection of blood from the left ventricle into the aorta and great vessels.

3. Carotid, radial, brachial, femoral, popliteal, dorsalis pedis, and posterior tibial pulses should be examined bilaterally.

4. Rate, rhythm, amplitude, and pulse contour are noted.

Grading of Arterial Pulses

0	Absent or found with doppler only
1+	Thready, fades in and out, easily obliterated with pressure
2+ (normal)	Palpable, less easily obliterated with pressure
3+	Easily palpated, not easily obliterated with pressure
4+	Bounding, often visible, not obliterated with pressure

5. Auscultation of carotid, abdominal aorta, and femoral arteries should be done to detect bruits or thrills.

6. Bruits or thrills are caused by an abnormal flow or turbulence of blood through an artery.

7. Bruits (blowing sounds) are best heard when the patient holds his/her breath.

8. Thrills are abnormal vibrations which may be felt over the arteries.

9. Pulse abnormalities include small, weak pulses; large, bounding pulses; water hammer or collapsing pulses; pulsus alternans; bigeminal pulse; pulsus paradoxus and pulsus bisferiens.

Small, Weak Pulses:
- Difficult to feel.
- May occur when there is partial arterial occlusion (proximal to the pulse) or whenever there is decreased cardiac output.
- May be present in shock or left ventricular failure when there is decreased stroke volume.
- Stenotic valves can also lead to diminished pulses because a mechanical obstruction is present.

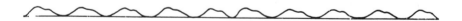

Mary Canobbio, *Cardiovascular Disorders*, Saint Louis: Mosby-Year Book, 1990. Used with permission of the publisher.

Large, Bounding Pulses:
- Readily palpable, as an increased stroke volume is generally present.
- Can occur in hyperkinetic states such as exercise, anxiety, fear, fever, anemia and hyperthyroidism.
- May also be present with increased aortic rigidity, as in aging and atherosclerosis.

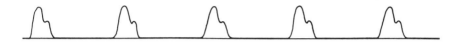

Mary Canobbio, *Cardiovascular Disorders*, Saint Louis: Mosby-Year Book, 1990. Used with permission of the publisher.

Water-hammer or Collapsing Pulse:
- Has a greater amplitude, rapid upstroke, high momentary peak and sudden downstroke.
- Classically associated with aortic insufficiency, and patent ductus.

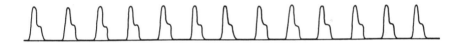

Mary Canobbio, *Cardiovascular Disorders*, Saint Louis: Mosby-Year Book, 1990. Used with permission of the publisher.

Pulsus Alternans:
- Characterized by alternate strong and weak pulse beats with a regular rhythm.
- May be an early sign of left ventricular failure.

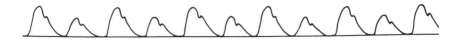

Mary Canobbio, *Cardiovascular Disorders*, Saint Louis: Mosby-Year Book, 1990. Used with permission of the publisher.

Bigeminal Pulse:

- Produced by changes in the volume of blood being ejected from the left ventricle.
- Rhythm is irregular and the arterial pulsations alternate in size from one beat to the next.
- Usually produced by a premature ventricular contraction (PVC) that occurs after a normally conducted beat.

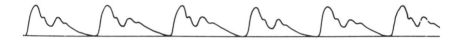

Mary Canobbio, *Cardiovascular Disorders*, Saint Louis: Mosby-Year Book, 1990. Used with permission of the publisher.

Pulsus Paradoxus:

- Characterized by a change of amplitude during respiration.
- Results in decreased amplitude during inspiration and increased amplitude during expiration.
- Heart rhythm and rate are unchanged.
- Associated with conditions that impair venous return (constrictive pericarditis, pericardial effusion, or cardiac tamponade).
- Commonly found in persons with asthma, emphysema or tracheal obstruction in which there is exaggerated respiratory movements of the ribs and diaphragm during inspiration to overcome a respiratory obstruction.

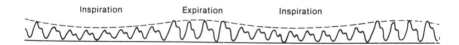

Mary Canobbio, *Cardiovascular Disorders*, Saint Louis: Mosby-Year Book, 1990. Used with permission of the publisher.

Pulsus Bisferiens:
- Seen in aortic stenosis and hypertrophic cardiomyopathy.

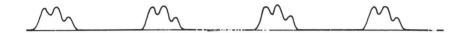

Mary Canobbio, *Cardiovascular Disorders*, **Saint Louis: Mosby-Year Book, 1990.
Used with permission of the publisher.**

Venous Pressures

1. Peripheral and central venous pressures give information regarding right-sided heart function.

2. Peripheral venous pressure is a constant pressure exerted by blood on the walls of veins.

3. Central venous pressure (CVP) indicates the pressure of or amount of blood in the right atrium.

4. Venous pressures may be determined directly or indirectly. (For discussion of direct methods, see Chapter 5.)

5. Indirect measurement of the peripheral venous pressure can be accomplished by inspection of the neck veins with the aid of a good light source.

6. Right internal jugular vein is preferred access site for measurement of CVP.

7. Pulsations and venous filling are present while the patient is lying flat.

8. As the head of the bed is elevated to 45°, the vein distension should disappear.

9. Bilateral jugular vein distension indicates increased CVP. Unilateral jugular vein distention may indicate a local vein blockage.

10. Sternal angle, or Angle of Louis, is used as a convenient bedside reference point for measuring venous pressure. It is located at the junction of the sternum with the second rib and lies approximately 5 cm above the right atrium (see **Figure 2.1**).

11. Venous distention is normally present when the head of the bed is less than 30°.

12. Pressures of more than 5 cm above the Angle of Louis reflect elevated right atrial pressure and may indicate right-sided heart failure.

   • Hepatojugular reflux is a phenomenon that indicates right-sided heart failure.

Technique to Determine Hepatojugular Reflux

♦ Patient is positioned so that highest venous pulsation is seen in the middle of the neck.
♦ Firm pressure is applied to patient's right upper quadrant for 30 to 60 seconds while patient breathes normally.
♦ Increase of greater than 1 cm is considered abnormal and an indication of right-sided heart failure.

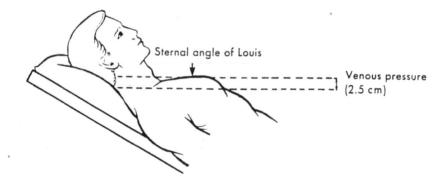

Sternal angle of Louis

Venous pressure (2.5 cm)

Figure 2.1. Venous pressure is estimated by measuring the vertical distance between the uppermost point of jugular pulsation and the Sternal Angle of Louis. Normally, this distance is less than 3 cm. M.R. Kinney, D.R. Packa, K.G. Andreoli, and D. P. Zipes, *Comprehensive Cardiac Care,*(7th edition) Saint Louis: Mosby-Year Book , 1991. Used with permission of the publisher.

Anatomy of the Heart

Location

1. The heart lies between the lungs in the middle of the thoracic cavity.

2. Two-thirds of the heart extends to the left of the body's midline.

3. The base of the heart faces up and to the right; the tip, or apex, faces down and to the left.

4. The heart is slightly rotated so that the right heart lies directly beneath the chest wall.

5. The apex is the small portion of the lower left ventricle that contracts during systole.

6. The precordium is the portion of the chest wall lying directly over the heart.

Chambers

1. The atria are thin-walled, and act as collecting chambers, or reservoirs, of systemic blood.

2. The ventricles are pumping chambers that send out blood to the body's tissues and lungs.

3. The left ventricle has a large, thick muscular wall that generates increased pressure to pump arterial blood into the systemic circulation.

Valves

1. The main function of the four cardiac valves is to ensure uni-directional blood flow through the cardiac circuit.

2. The tricuspid and mitral valves are known as atrioventricular valves (AV) and separate the atria from the ventricles.

3. The pulmonic and aortic valves are known as semilunar valves and separate the ventricles from the great vessels.

Examination of the Heart

1. **Inspection of the precordium:**

   a. Patient should be supine with the head of the bed elevated to approximately 30°.

b. Note the presence of the apical impulse or point of maximal impulse (PMI), the thrusting of the left ventricle against the chest wall. It is usually present in the 5th intercostal space (5ICS) at or just medial to the midclavicular line (MCL).

c. Inspect the entire precordium for visible lifting of the chest wall, called heaves or lifts, which are due to abnormally forceful cardiac action.

d. Inspection should be done in an orderly fashion: from aortic to pulmonic; third left interspace (Erb's point) to right ventricular or tricuspid area; and apical or mitral area to epigastric area (see **Figure 2.2**).

e. Note any abnormal pulsations which may be indicative of an aneurysm.

2. **Palpation of the precordium**:

  a. Utilize the same systematic approach as described for inspection.

  b. Palpate for heaves, pulsations and thrills (vibratory sensations produced by turbulent blood flow or forcing of blood through narrowed valves).

  c. Begin at base of the heart and palpate all areas using the palmar surface of the hand. The tips of the fingers may be used to more finely locate any findings.

  d. Palpate the apical impulse. Note its presence, location, size, and character. The amplitude may be increased in the thin-walled individual or when the patient is on his left side. It is felt in only half the population.

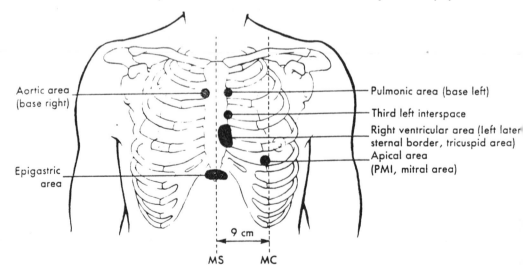

Aortic area (base right) — Pulmonic area (base left) — Third left interspace — Right ventricular area (left lateral sternal border, tricuspid area) — Apical area (PMI, mitral area) — Epigastric area — 9 cm — MS — MC

Figure 2.2. Inspection and palpation areas on the precordium for detecting normal and abnormal cardiac pulsations. M.R. Kinney, D.R. Packa, K.G. Andreoli, and D. P. Zipes, *Comprehensive Cardiac Care,* (7th edition) Saint Louis: Mosby-Year Book, 1991. Used with permission of the publisher.

Summary of Abnormal Findings on Inspection and Palpation

Precordium	Abnormality	Possible Causes
Aortic area (2ICS[‡], RSB[‡])	Forceful pulsation	Rheumatic heart disease; systemic hypertension; ascending thoracic aortic aneurysm
	Vibratory thrill	Aortic stenosis (AS)
Pulmonic area (2ICS[‡],LSB[‡])	Forceful pulsation	Pulmonary hypertension; left ventricular failure; mitral stenosis
Third left interspace or Erb's point (3ICS[‡], LSB[‡])	Vibratory thrill	Aortic or pulmonic valve diseases
Right ventricular or tricuspid area (4ICS[‡]LSB[‡])	Thrill	Ventricular septal defect (VSD)
	Heave or lift	Mitral stenosis (MS)
	Abnormal pulsation	Right ventricular enlargement
Apical or mitral area (5ICS[‡], LMCL[‡])	Strong apical impulse	Left ventricular hypertrophy; aortic valve diseases
	Dyskinetic apical impulse	Left ventricular aneurysm
	Thrill	Mitral valve disease
Epigastric area (the upper central region of the abdomen)	Strong pulsation	Abdominal aortic aneurysm; aortic valvular regurgitation
	Pulsation of liver	Congestive heart failure

‡ Key:
ICS—intercostal space; RSB—right sternal border; LSB—left sternal border and LMCL—left midclavicular line

3. **Percussion of the precordium:**

   a. Percussion is done to determine the left cardiac border.

   b. The fifth, fourth, and third intercostal spaces should be percussed sequentially until cardiac dullness is noted.

    c. Percussion is of limited value on the right side of the chest as the heart lies beneath the sternum.

    d. Cannot be done in obese patients, those with overdeveloped musculature, those with large breasts or advanced emphysema.

4. **Auscultation**:

    a. Enables the practitioner to evaluate cardiac rate, rhythm, normal and abnormal heart sounds.

    b. Rate should be counted for one full minute.

    c. Rhythm should be identified as regular or irregular. If irregular, note any pattern.

    d. Heart sounds result from the opening and closing of valves and the flow of blood through the heart during the normal cardiac cycle.

    e. The diaphragm of the stethoscope is used to listen to high-pitched sounds such as the first and second heart sounds.

    f. The bell of the stethoscope, when applied lightly to the chest wall, is used for low-pitched sounds such as the third and fourth heart sounds and murmurs.

    g. Complete auscultatory examination should be conducted with the patient in a supine, left-lateral, and sitting position.

    h. A systematic approach should be used to auscultate for normal and abnormal heart sounds at the five most common cardiac areas.

    i. The five auscultatory areas are similar to the inspection and palpation areas and are located as follows (See **Figure 2.2** on page 36.):

      • Aortic valve area: second intercostal space at the right sternal border (2ICS,RSB).

      • Pulmonic valve area: second intercostal space at the left sternal border (2ICS,LSB).

      • Third intercostal space at the left sternal border or Erb's point (3ICS,LSB).

      • Tricuspid area: fourth intercostal space along the lower left sternal border (4ICS,LSB).

      • Mitral (or apical) area: fifth intercostal space at the left midclavicular line (5ICS,LMCL).

    j. There are four basic heart sounds S_1, S_2, S_3, and S_4. The detection of normal and extra heart sounds is detailed in **Table 2.1** on the pages 39 40 and 41.

Table 2.1. Heart Sounds

Heart Sounds	Etiology	Location	Quality	Clinical Conditions
S₁ (**lub** of lub-dub)	Closure of tricuspid and mitral valves synchronous with apical impulse and corresponds to contraction of ventricles or systole.	Apical or mitral area (5ICS, LMCL)	High-pitch (diaphragm)	
Splitting of S₁ "**T-lub**-dub"	Mitral valve closes slightly before tricuspid valve, due to asynchronous contraction of left and right ventricles.	Tricuspid area (4ICS, LSB)	High-pitch (diaphragm)	
S₂ (the **dub** of lub-dub)	Closure of the aortic and pulmonic valves, corresponds to ventricular diastole.	Aortic area or base (2ICS, RSB)	High-pitch (diaphragm)	
Splitting of S₂ "lub-t-**dub**"	Exaggerated during inspiration due to slight asynchrony of aortic and pulmonary valve closure.	Pulmonic area (2ICS, LSB)	High-pitch (diaphragm)	

Heart Sounds	Etiology	Location	Quality	Clinical Conditions
S₃ "ventricular gallop" "y" in "Ken-tuck-y" or "lub-dub-**dee**"	Rapid filling of ventricle in early diastole.	Apical or mitral area (5ICS, LMCL)	Low-pitch (Bell)	Early sign of failure. Ventricular aneurysm. Common in young adults and children.
S₄ "atrial gallop" "**dee**-lub-dub" or "**ten**-nes-see"	Occurs in late diastole, following atrial contraction. Atria make extra effort to fill against resistance.	Apical or mitral area (5ICS, LMCL)	Low-pitch (Bell)	Occurs with left ventricular hypertrophy due to HTN, CAD, AV disease and cardiomyopathy. Aortic stenosis.
Summation gallop	S₃ and S₄ fuse with rapid heart rates. Diastole is shortened. Early and late ventricular filling phases coincide.	Apical or mitral area (5ICS, LMCL)	Low-pitch (Bell)	Tachycardia and severe myocardial disease.
Opening snap	Occurs in early diastole after the second heart sound.	Apical or mitral area (5ICS, LMCL)	High-pitch (diaphragm)	Mitral or tricuspid stenosis.

Heart Sounds	Etiology	Location	Quality	Clinical Conditions
Systolic click (systolic ejection sound)	Heard immediately after S_1. Associated with valvular or great vessel vibrations.	Apical or mitral area (5ICS, LMCL)	High pitch (diaphragm)	Mitral valve prolapse. Aortic stenosis. Aneurysms of the ascending aorta, congenital bicuspid aortic valve, systemic hypertension.
		Pulmonic area (2ICS, LSB)	High-pitch (diaphragm)	Pulmonary hypertension. Pulmonary stenosis.
Pericardial friction rub	Rubbing of visceral and parietal pericardium.	Third left interspace at the left sternal border or Erbs point (3ICS, LSB)	High-pitch (diaphragm)	Pericardial inflammation.

Murmurs

Murmurs are vibrations or abnormal sounds caused by turbulent blood flow through the heart or great vessels. (See **Table 2.2** on page 44 for common heart murmurs.) They are transmitted to the surface of the chest.

- Murmurs are usually associated with valvular dysfunction, septal defects, or loose structures which can vibrate.
- Murmurs identified in cardiac assessment should be classified according to the following six characteristics. These include:
  - Timing or occurrence in cardiac cycle
  - Location
  - Intensity
  - Quality
  - Pitch
  - Radiation

1. **Timing or occurrence in cardiac cycle:**

   a. Murmurs are timed according to the phase of the cardiac cycle in which they occur.

   b. Systolic murmurs can occur in early, middle, or late systole. They are audible between S_1 and S_2, and they coincide with the apical pulse.

   c. Mid-systolic ejection murmurs begin after the first sound, swell to a crescendo in mid-systole, then decrease in intensity, and terminate before S_2.

   d. Holosystolic murmurs last throughout ventricular systole.

   e. Diastolic murmurs occur in early, middle, or late diastole.

2. **Location:**

   a. The area on the precordium where the intensity of the murmur is greatest should be identified.

   b. Murmurs that are valvular in origin are usually heard best over their respective valve areas. This is not directly over the valve, but rather over the area where the blood is ejected. Sound travels in the direction of ejection.

3. **Intensity:**

   a. Assess the loudness of the murmur.

   b. The intensity of a murmur is generally described using a grading scale of 1-6 as follows:

Grade I	Very faint
Grade II	Faint, but distinct
Grade III	Moderately loud
Grade IV	Loud, associated with a thrill
Grade V	Very loud, thrill easily palpable
Grade VI	Audible without stethoscope, thrill palpable

4. **Quality**:

   a. The quality describes the tonal characteristic of the murmur.

   b. Quality may be described as blowing, rumbling, harsh or musical.

   c. A crescendo murmur is one that increases in intensity after its onset.

   d. A decrescendo murmur is one that decreases in intensity after its onset.

   e. A crescendo-decrescendo or diamond-shaped murmur is one that first increases and then decreases.

5. **Pitch:**

   a. The pitch is the sound frequency of the murmur.

   b. It is classified as high, medium or low.

6. **Radiation**:

   a. Transmission or radiation of the murmur to other parts of the body should be indicated.

   b. The sound may radiate to the head, neck, axilla, back or extremities.

Table 2.2. Common Heart Murmurs

Timing	Etiology	Location	Quality	Pitch	Radiation
Pansystolic/ Holosystolic (systole)	Mitral regurgitation (MR)	Mitral area	Blowing	High	Left axilla
	Tricuspid regurgitation (TR)	Tricuspid area	Blowing	High	Toward apex
	Ventricular septal defect (VSD)	Lower left sternal border	Harsh	High	Precordium
Mid-systolic (Crescendo/ Decrescendo)	Aortic stenosis (AS)	Aortic area	Harsh	High	Carotids
	Pulmonic stenosis (PS)	Pulmonic area	Harsh	High	Lower LSB and toward left shoulder and neck
Early diastolic (Decrescendo)	Aortic regurgitation (AR)	3 or 4ICS	Blowing	High	LSB
	Pulmonic regurgitation (PR)	Left sternal border	Blowing	High	
Mid-to-late diastolic (Crescendo/ Decrescendo)	Mitral stenosis (MS)	Apical/Mitral area	Rumbling	Low	None
	Tricuspid stenosis (TS)	Lower left sternal border	Rumbling	Low-Medium	None

Selected References

Bates, B. *A Guide to Physical Examination.* (5th edition) Philadelphia: J.B. Lippincott Company, 1990.

Canobbio, Mary. *Cardiovascular Disorders.* Saint Louis: Mosby-Year Book, 1990.

Epstein, E.J. *Cardiac Auscultation.* Oxford: Butterworth-Heinemann Ltd., 1991.

Guzzetta, C., and Dossey, B.M. *Cardiovascular Nursing—Bodymind Tapestry.* (2nd edition) Saint Louis: The C.V. Mosby Company, 1992.

Kinney, M.R., Packa, D.R., Andreoli, K.G., and Zipes, D.P. *Comprehensive Cardiac Care.* (7th edition) Saint Louis: Mosby-Year Book, Inc., 1991.

Seidel, H., Ball, J.W., Dains, J.E., and Benedict, G.W. *Mosby's Guide to Physical Examination.* (2nd edition) St. Louis: Mosby-Year Book, Inc., 1991.

CHAPTER THREE

PRINCIPLES OF PRESSURE TRANSDUCER MONITORING

A basic understanding of the technical components of the hemodynamic monitoring equipment is essential to the practitioner to ensure accurate readings. This chapter will review these technical components. The four components of any hemodynamic system are a transducer, an amplifier, a display instrument, and a catheter/tubing system.

Transducer/Amplifier

1. The transducer detects pressure changes from within the cannulated vessel and transmits that energy to the amplifier system.

2. The conversion of the physiological event to an electrical signal occurs by displacement of a diaphragm within the transducer.

3. The amplifier detects this electrical change in the transducer and amplifies it while filtering out interference.

System Set Up

◆ Wash hands.
◆ Turn on monitor.
◆ Prepare heparinized saline:
  — Remove all air from saline bag by inverting the bag and inserting a needle in the medication port.
◆ Assemble pressure tubing and transducer set-up. Make certain all connections are tightened.
NOTE: Most institutions use pre-assembled kits.
◆ Spike heparinized saline bag, fill drip chamber to point and flush.
◆ Flush out all stopcocks maintaining sterility of the system including all caps.
◆ Replace vented caps with sterile dead-ender caps.
◆ Apply pressure bag and pump up to 300 mm Hg.
◆ Attach system to transducer holder.
◆ Connect transducer to the amplifier/monitor system.

Balancing

Accuracy of pressure readings is based on correct leveling or balancing of the transducer.

1. The transducer air-fluid interface (the open stopcock), should be level with the catheter's distal tip. When arterial pressure is being monitored, the transducer must be leveled with the cannulated artery. Intrathoracic pressure monitoring requires leveling at the right atrium or phlebostatic axis. This is measured at the fourth intercostal space at the mid axillary line (**Figure. 3.1**).

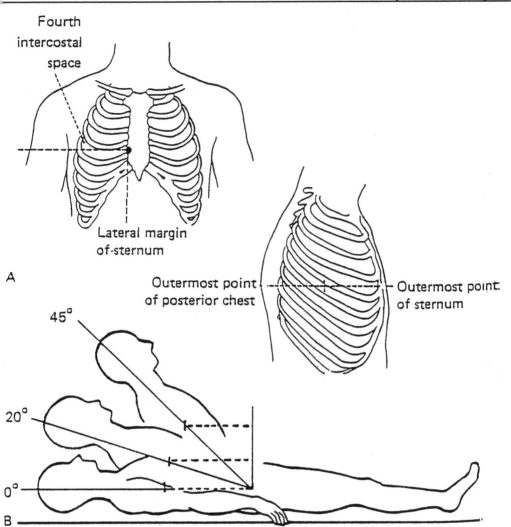

Fourth
intercostal
space

Lateral margin
of-sternum

A

Outermost point
of posterior chest

Outermost point
of sternum

45°

20°

0°

B

Figure 3.1. The phlebostatic axis is the crossing of two reference lines: a line
from the fourth intercostal space at a point where it joins the sternum, drawn out
to the side beneath the axilla, and a line midpoint between the anterior and
posterior surfaces of the chest. Maxine Patrick, Susan Woods, Ruth Craven,
Joanne Schnaidt Rokosky, and Pauline Bruno, *Medical Surgical Nursing:
Pathophysiological Concepts*, Philadelphia: J.B. Lippincott, 1994. Used with permission of the publisher.

2. Utilize a carpenter's level to ensure accurate leveling of the transducer stopcock with the catheter's distal tip. This will eliminate the effect of the hydrostatic forces. If the transducer is placed too high, the resulting reading will be falsely low. Conversely, if the transducer is placed too low, the resultant readings will be falsely high. A change in position of either patient or transducer by one inch is equivalent to approximately 2 mm Hg change in pressure. Remember, the actual pressure has not changed, just the measured numbers. If the transducer and/or patient position has changed, this procedure should be performed before each reading.

Leveling/Balancing

- Position the patient supine so the patient and bed are in the 0-45° position.
- Locate the zero reference point—the position of the catheter tip.
  - Intrathoracic Pressures:
    - Palpate the 4th intercostal space along the sternum and extend laterally.
    - Locate mid-axillary line—halfway between the anterior and posterior chest.
    - Locate the point at which the two lines intersect.
  - Arterial Pressures:
    - Locate the position of the catheter tip.
- Mark this level on the patient.
- Utilizing a carpenter's level, mount the transducer on a pole, so the air-fluid interface is level with the reference point.

NOTE: The transducer may be mounted directly on the patient.

Zero Reference

Before patient pressures are monitored, the transducer must be given a zero reference point. The reference point is atmospheric pressure. When the nurse opens the stopcock (off to patient and open to air) between the patient and transducer (usually the stopcock attached to the transducer), the pressures on either side of the transducer diaphragm equalize. The diaphragm will not send signals to the amplifier/monitor because the diaphragm is flat. The amplifier/monitor should then read zero. All pressures applied to the transducer after this point will be referenced to this zero.

Zeroing

+ Open the stopcock on the transducer by turning it off to the patient and open to air. (Remove dead-ender cap maintaining sterility.)
+ Adjust the monitor so the digital display reads zero.
+ Turn the stopcock so it is open to patient and closed to air.
+ Replace sterile dead-ender cap.
NOTE: The zero function on each monitor is different. Consult the instruction manual.

Catheter/Tubing System

The system is comprised of an indwelling catheter which connects to fluid-filled pressure tubing. (Refer to **Figure 3.2.**)

1. Fluid transmits impulses to the transducer.

2. To maintain patency of this fluid-filled system, normal saline with heparin will be placed under 300 mm Hg continuous pressure via a pressure bag. Under certain circumstances the physician may elect not to put heparin in the bag. (Note: The usual heparin dose is 2 units/ml.)

3. A flush device in the set-up provides a continuous flush of about 3 cc per hour and allows for manual flushing when necessary. This prevents the backflow of blood which may clot off the catheter and/or alter the pressure waveform.

4. Non-distensible pressure tubing is utilized to prevent distortion of the waveform. Compliant tubing distorts the waveform by absorbing energy and sending it back to the system some time later.

5. Keeping non-distensible tubing length to a minimum also ensures greater accuracy in the waveform.

6. Stopcocks are utilized throughout the system to allow for blood sampling and zeroing of the transducer.

7. Frequency response and damping coefficient are characteristics of the tubing system which affect the accuracy of the pressure waveform.

8. "The frequency response refers to the system's ability to reproduce all of the waveform components being generated" (Ahrens, T. and Taylor, L. 1992, p. 212). Frequency response measures the oscillations in Hertz or cycles per second. Acceptable frequency response for hemodynamic equipment is ½ Hz to 40 Hz. Manufacturers of hemodynamic equipment usually ensure that the frequency response is adequate for hemodynamic waveform reproduction.

9. The damping coefficient is the "ability to reproduce the changes in the actual waveform." (Ahrens, T. and Taylor, L. 1992, p. 213).

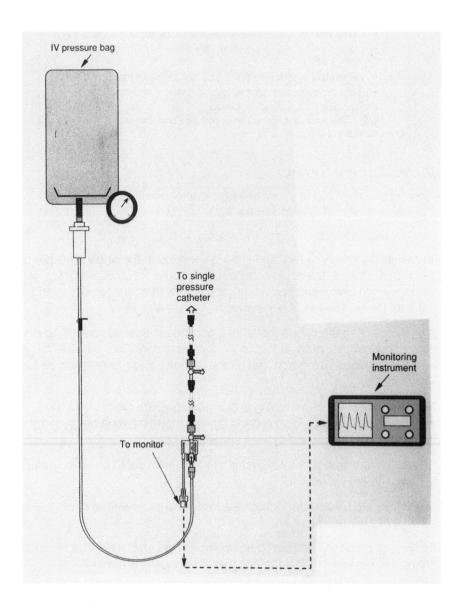

Figure 3.2. Pressure monitoring system. Photo courtesy of Baxter Healthcare Corporation, Edwards Critical-Care Division. Used with permission.

10. In combination they act to produce an accurate waveform. The damping coefficient is much like a shock absorber. If the system is underdamped, the waveform will have large oscillations. If the system is overdamped, there will be loss of oscillations.

11. To test the frequency response, perform a square wave test. For the specific procedure please refer to Chapter 4.

Calibration

Calibration is the procedure of introducing a known pressure into the system and ensuring the transducer accurately reads this pressure. Although transducer calibration should be performed prior to the initiation of hemodynamic monitoring, widespread use of disposable transducers has limited this practice. Some manufacturers provide a device which can be connected to the system for the purpose of introducing a known pressure. The practitioner must be certain to maintain sterility of the system during this procedure.

Table 3.1. Monitoring Problems

Problem	Causes	Interventions
No waveform	• Stopcocks in off position • Monitor not on proper scale • Monitor not functioning • Transducer not functioning • Completely kinked catheter • Completely clotted catheter • Patient asystolic	• Open all stopcocks • Check scales • Replace monitor • Replace transducer • Check for kinks • Aspirate clot • ACLS protocol
Dampened waveform	• Air bubble/blood in line • Clot at catheter tip • Disconnected or loose tubing • Underinflated pressure bag • Catheter tip against wall • Compliant tubing	• Flush air/blood from system • Aspirate clot • Tighten all connections • Reinflate bag to 300 mm Hg • Reposition catheter • Replace with pressure tubing
Underdamped waveform	• Too many stopcocks • Long tubing • Tiny air bubbles • Defective transducer	• Limit stopcocks • Shorten tubing • Flush air from system • Replace transducer

The above chart is a summary of common monitoring problems, their causes and corrective interventions.

Selected References

Aherns, T., and Taylor, L. *Hemodynamic Waveform Analysis.* Philadelphia: W.B. Saunders, 1992.

Baxter-Edwards. *Invasive Hemodynamic Monitoring: Physiologic Principles and Clinical Applications.* California: Baxter Healthcare Corporation, 1989.

Dennison, R.D. "Making sense of hemodynamic monitoring." *AJN*, 94(8) 24-32, 1994.

Gardner, P. "Pulmonary artery pressure monitoring." *AACN Clinical Issues in Critical Care Nursing*, 4 (1), 98-119, 1993.

Kern, L. "Hemodynamic monitoring." *AACN Procedure Manual for Critical Care.* (3rd edition) Philadelphia: W.B. Saunders Company, 1993.

McIntire, B. "Troubleshooting invasive hemodynamic monitoring systems. " *Critical Care Choices,* 43-46, 1993.

CHAPTER FOUR

TECHNIQUES OF INVASIVE ARTERIAL PRESSURE MONITORING

Invasive blood pressure monitoring is the cannulation of an artery and the attachment of the catheter to high pressure, fluid filled tubing. The pressure in the system is converted into a digital electrical signal and displayed on an oscilloscope.

Indications for Invasive Blood Pressure Monitoring

- To continuously monitor arterial blood pressure in the setting of unstable states associated with hypotension and decreased cardiac output. In low-flow states, decreased pulsatile flow will obscure Korotkoff sounds making the cuff pressure an unreliable method of blood pressure monitoring.
- To continuously monitor arterial blood pressure in altered states associated with excessive vasoconstriction.
- To monitor the effects of vasoactive medications, both hypotensive and hypertensive agents. Beat to beat systolic, diastolic, and mean pressures provide rapid assessment of therapy.
- To provide an easy access for frequent arterial blood sampling.

Insertion Sites

1. Criteria for selection are as follows:

   - Vessel should be large so that the catheter will not occlude the lumen.
   - Artery should have collateral circulation.
   - Catheter should have easy access for care.
   - Area should not be prone to contamination.

2. The radial, axillary, femoral, and dorsal pedal arteries are sites for cannulation. Each of the above sites has advantages and disadvantages associated with cannulation (**Table 4.2**). In practice in critical care units, the radial and femoral arteries are most commonly used for arterial monitoring. Before the dorsal pedal artery is cannulated, collateral circulation through the posterior tibial artery should be demonstrated.

To test for collateral circulation to the hand from the ulnar artery, the Modified Allen test must be performed (**Table 4.1**). Delays of greater than 15 - 20 seconds or absence of return of color indicate that the artery should not be used for cannulation.

Table 4.1. Modified Allen Test

- ◆ Elevate the patient's arm above the level of the heart.
- ◆ Have the patient open and close his hand several times, then tightly clench his fist.
- ◆ Occlude both the radial and ulnar arteries.
- ◆ Lower the patient's hand and unclench fist while still holding pressure on the radial artery.
- ◆ Observe for return of color to the hand within 7 seconds.

Table 4.2. Most Common Complications of Arterial Cannulation

Artery	Common Complications	Other Complications
Radial	⊛ Ischemia and necrosis secondary to thrombosis and embolism	
Femoral		A-V fistula/false aneurysm
Axillary	⊛ Hemorrhage	Neurological */‡
Dorsal Pedal	⊛ Infection	

*Patients on anticoagulant therapy may have subfascial bleeding which leads to median nerve neuropathy and contraction of the fingers and/or wrist with loss of power.

‡Axillary sheath hematoma may lead to nerve compression.

Pressure Wave Physiology

For a review of the factors affecting arterial blood pressure see Chapter One.

1. Blood is rapidly ejected during systole from the left ventricle into the aorta, causing the walls of the aorta to stretch and the pressure to rise.

2. The aorta acts as a reservoir and most of the ejected blood is accommodated by stretching the walls of the aorta. The ejected blood does not reach the peripheral arteries until several heartbeats later.

3. The stretch is converted to potential energy to permit a continuous flow of blood even during diastole. This stretch initiates a pressure curve that is dispersed along the aorta and its branches.

4. It is the pressure wave that one palpates, as the pulse, in various arterial locations on the body.

5. Arterial pressure waves change in shape as they travel away from the aorta (**Figure 4.1**).

   These changes are pronounced in young individuals but diminish with age. The changes are as follows:

   a. Delay occurs in the time of onset of the initial pressure rise

   b. The sharp incisura or dicrotic notch dampens out and is less pronounced.

   c. The systolic portion of the pressure curve becomes narrowed and tall.

   d. Systolic pressure increases, diastolic pressure decreases slightly, and mean arterial pressure remains unchanged or decreases slightly as the pulse travels away from the heart. These changes produce little effect to the circulation, but it is important to remember whenever arterial pressure is monitored peripherally. Normally, systolic blood pressure is 20-30 mm Hg higher in the legs than in the arms.

6. The speed of transmission of the pulse is determined by the compliance of the vessel. Atherosclerosis which decreases compliance increases the speed of transmission. With aging, there are changes in the collagen and elastin contents of the arterial walls which decrease aortic compliance; the heart is less able to eject its stroke volume rapidly into the aorta.

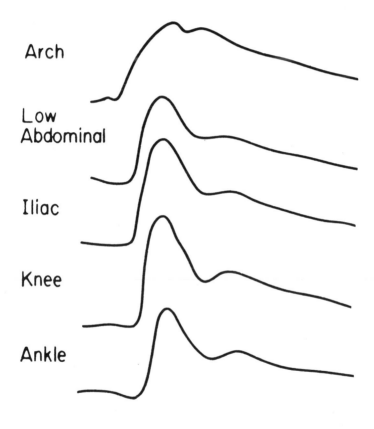

Arch

Low
Abdominal

Iliac

Knee

Ankle

Figure 4.1. Arterial pressure curves from various sites.

Pressure Wave Contour

1. The arterial pressure waveform is divided into systole and diastole (Refer to Chapter One for additional information and **Figure 1.4**).

2. During ventricular systole, blood is ejected into the aorta and causes an increase in pressure. The highest pressure of the pressure wave is the **systolic pressure (Figure 4.2)**.

3. After systole, even after the ventricular pressure falls, the elastic stretch of arterial walls maintains high pressure in the arteries.

4. As the blood moves downstream, the pressure falls and is noted by the sharp decline on the pressure curve.

5. This sharp downward pressure drop is followed by the upward deflection known as the **dicrotic notch** or **incisura (Figure 4.2)**. This notch denotes the end of systole and the beginning of diastole. The dicrotic notch is caused by the backward flow of blood from the aorta toward the ventricle causing the aortic valve to close.

6. This is followed by a slow pressure decline back to the diastolic level. The lowest pressure on the pressure wave is the **diastolic pressure.**

7. The difference between the systolic and diastolic pressure is the **pulse** pressure. It is a function of stroke volume and arterial capacitance.

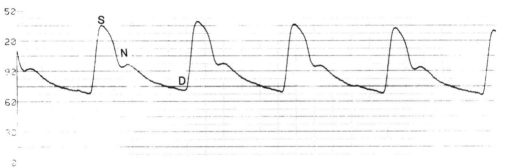

Figure 4.2. Normal arterial pressure wave contour. The normal contour has a sharp upstroke, clear dicrotic notch, and a definite end diastolic point.
S = systole
D = diastole
N = dicrotic notch

8. **Mean arterial pressure** (MAP) represents the average of the two pressures during the cardiac cycle. It depends only on the cardiac output and systemic vascular resistance. The calculation of MAP = diastolic pressure + 1/3 pulse pressure. Another method of calculation of the MAP = (1 systole + 2 diastole) /3. Normal values are between 70-105 mm Hg (see appendix).

According to the laws of physics, pressure is equal to flow times resistance (see Chapter One for further discussion). That formula can be restated as MAP = CO (milliliters/minute) × SVR (millimeters Hg/milliliter/minute).

Therefore, blood pressure is affected by cardiac output and peripheral resistance. The manipulation of any one of these variables will ultimately affect the others.

9. The beginning of ventricular systole coincides with the peak of the R wave. The rapid rise occurs immediately after the QRS complex (**Figure 4.3**). When observing this on a paper tracing, the nurse may observe a delay of 0.2 seconds after the end of the QRS. The amount of delay will depend upon the location of the peripheral catheter. The dicrotic notch occurs after the T wave of the EKG.

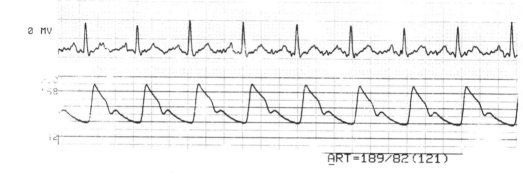

Figure 4.3. Normal sinus rhythm with arterial blood pressure waveform. The EKG tracing has artifact. Notice the beginning of ventricular systole coincides with the peak of the R wave and the rapid rise of the waveform occurs immediately after the QRS complex. The dicrotic notch occurs after the T wave.

EKG Correlations with Arterial Blood Pressure Waves

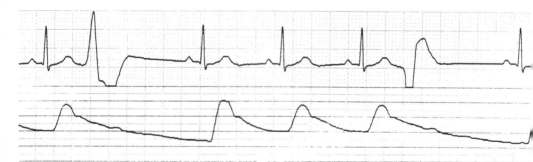

Figure 4.4. Normal sinus rhythm with premature ventricular contraction. Note the loss of blood pressure with the ectopic beats. This is due to loss of synchrony between the atrium and the ventricle. The loss of atrial contribution can decrease stroke volume up to 30%. In addition, these ectopic beats were early in diastole probably before the completion of rapid ventricular filling.

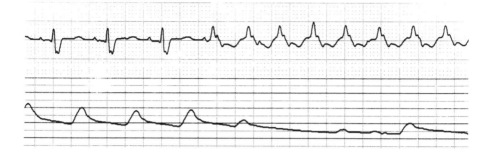

Figure 4.5. Ventricular tachycardia. This patient is pulseless as noted by the loss of arterial blood pressure.

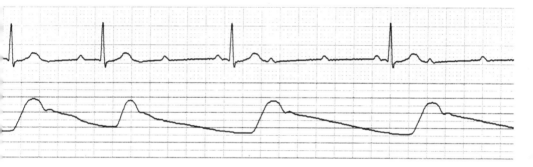

Figure 4.6. Second degree heart block, type I-Wenckebach to second degree heart block, type II. There is a dropped QRS complex and a corresponding loss of arterial blood pressure waveform.

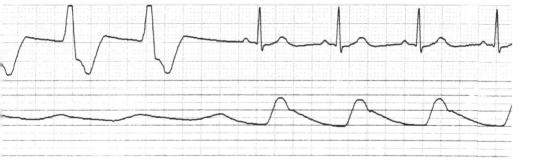

Figure 4.7. Accelerated idioventricular rhythm changing to normal sinus rhythm. The arterial blood pressure waveform of the accelerated idioventricular rhythm is slow to rise due to a decreased stroke volume. With the conversion to sinus rhythm and normal diastolic filling, the blood pressure increases.

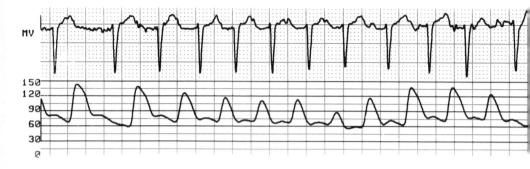

Figure 4.8. Atrial fibrillation. The blood pressure varies depending upon the R to R intervals. The shorter the R to R intervals, the less time for ventricular filling. In atrial fibrillation, there is loss of synchrony between the atria and the ventricles which also decreases blood pressure. This waveform is dampened and needs to be flushed.

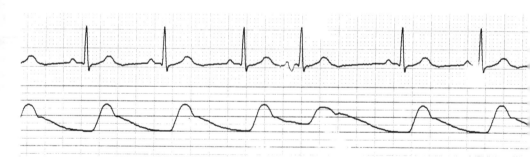

Figure 4.9. Normal sinus rhythm with a premature atrial contraction. Note the modest decrease in blood pressure with the ectopic beats. This is due to a shortened diastolic filling time and, therefore, a decreased stroke volume.

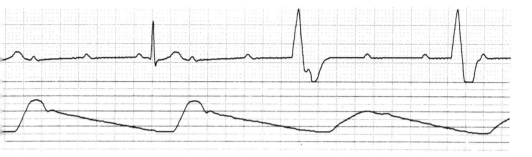

Figure 4.10. Second to third degree heart block. Notice the decrease in blood pressure as the rhythm changes from second to third degree heart block. In second degree heart block, there is a loss of blood pressure with the dropped beat, but there is normal ventricular filling. In third degree heart block, there is atrial/ventricular dissociation with loss of atrial filling.

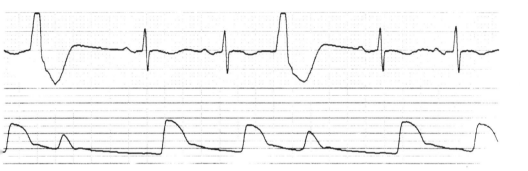

Figure 4.11. Dampened waveform. The contour is rounded and without a dicrotic notch. Aspiration and flushing may improve this tracing. Note the decreased blood pressure with the ectopic premature ventricular beats.

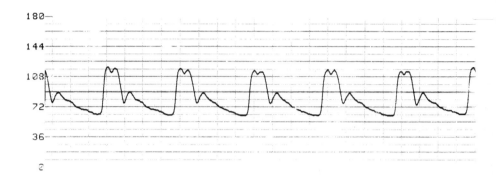

Figure 4.12. Pulsus bisferiens or double peaked pulse. This is most often seen in patients with hypertrophic cardiomyopathy. There is a rapid ejection of blood into the aorta, a slight decline in pressure due to the obstruction, and then a small pressure rise during continued ventricular systole.

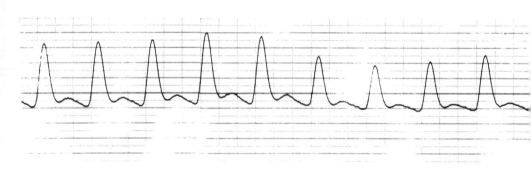

← Inspiration→   ←Expiration →

Figure 4.13. Patient on a positive pressure ventilator and hypovolemic. Note the exaggerated rise (10 mm Hg) of arterial blood pressure during inspiration. There is loss of dicrotic notch.

Invasive Versus Non-invasive Blood Pressure Monitoring

1. Check the accuracy of the invasive with the noninvasive method of blood pressure monitoring (**Table 4.3**).

2. Invasive pressure is always higher than cuff measurement. Expect a variance of 5 to 20 mm Hg. Refer to pressure wave physiology for further explanation.

3. Disparity may be due to incorrect cuff size and placement as well as improper calibration or "zeroing."

4. When noninvasive pressure is greater than invasive pressure, consider equipment malfunction or technical error. Refer to Chapter Three for possible sources of error.

5. Large variances of greater than 20-30 mm Hg may occur in patients with conditions causing vasoconstriction.

6. When all the equipment and tubing has been checked and is functioning satisfactorily and the discrepancy still exists, then the physiological condition of the patient needs to be considered. **In states which decrease flow to the periphery, invasive blood pressure monitoring is more accurate.**

Table 4.3. Evaluation of Blood Pressure

- Place bladder of blood pressure cuff over the brachial artery on the same arm as the cannulated artery.
- Inflate cuff until blood pressure waveform is no longer on the oscilloscope.
- Release cuff slowly until arterial waveform reappears.
- Note the mercury and gauge readings when the waveform reappears. This is the systolic blood pressure.

Technique for comparison of invasive/noninvasive blood pressure measurement. Do not assume the cuff pressure is more accurate because you heard it "with your ears."

Arterial Blood Pressure Monitoring Equipment

The components of this system are the same as for other invasive lines. Refer to Chapter Three and **Figure 4.14** for a complete description of the equipment, calibration, zeroing and troubleshooting techniques.

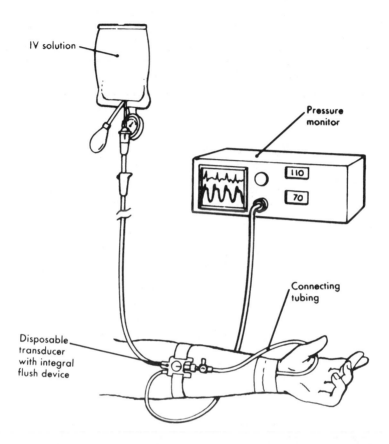

Figure 4.14. Example of the radial artery being used for arterial pressure monitoring with components of tubing, solution, transducer and pressure module.
Elaine Daily and John Schroeder, *Techniques in Bedside Hemodynamic Monitoring* **(5th edition) Saint Louis: Mosby-Year Book, 1994. Used with permission of the publisher.**

To measure the natural frequency and damping coefficient of the system and to ensure accurate waveforms, a snap-test or fast-flush should be done:

- At least once per shift (at the beginning of each shift for baseline)
- Whenever the system is opened
- Whenever the pressure waveform appears dampened.

Activate the fast flush feature on the fluid line. The test will produce a square wave pressure tracing followed by 2-3 oscillations before returning to the pressure waveform. This characteristic pattern is noted in **Figure 4.15**.

Overdamped response represents a loss of physiological signals in the system. This produces a square wave which does not fall below baseline and the fast-flush release does not produce an oscillatory response (**Figure 4.15**). Overdamped responses produce falsely low systolic and falsely high diastolic readings. The overdamped waveform produces a slow upstroke, narrow pulse pressure, and a loss of the dicrotic notch.

Underdamped responses produce wide variations above and below the baseline before oscillations return to normal morphology (**Figure 4.15**). They produce falsely high systolic and low diastolic readings. Underdamped responses have peaked systolic waves and prominent dicrotic notches.

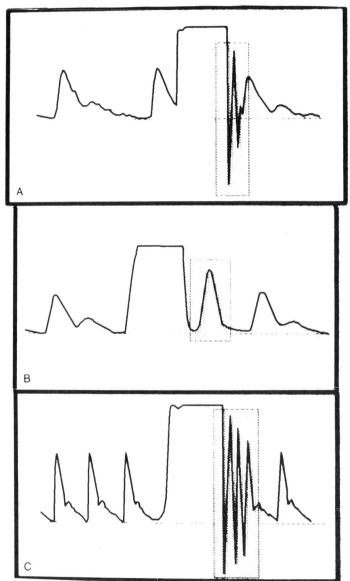

Figure 4.15. Square wave contour using the fast-flush feature on the hemodynamic fluid line. A, accurate waveform; B, overdamped; C, underdamped. See text for details. Courtesy of Baxter Healthcare Corporation, Edwards Critical-Care Division. Used with permission.

Caring for a Patient with an Arterial Line

Site

1. Immobilize site of cannulation.

2. Use Luer Locks to prevent accidental dislodgement and exsanguination.

3. Keep cannulation site visible to prevent exsanguination.

4. Track date of catheter insertion. Adhere to Center for Disease Control guidelines and/or hospital policy for specifics concerning catheter.

5. Change arterial line dressing in accordance with hospital policy.

6. Observe site for signs of infection or other complications every shift (at the beginning of the shift for baseline).

7. Assess circulation, sensation, and movement distal to insertion site every 2 hours.

Equipment

1. Use only high pressure tubing from insertion site to transducer (see Chapter Three). Change lines every 48-72 hours or in accordance with hospital policy. Avoid kinks in lines.

2. Assess accuracy of arterial waveform on oscilloscope continuously.

3. Troubleshoot any problems with dampened waveforms and variations in cuff versus invasive arterial blood pressure.

4. Document waveform with scale every shift and with significant changes.

5. Record systolic, diastolic and MAP according to unit protocol.

6. Set alarms

Blood Sampling

There are various methods for obtaining blood samples from an arterial line. See **Table 4.4** for one method. There are "bloodless" systems available which return the potentially discarded blood back to the patient. In these setups, there is a reservoir into which the aspirated blood would be held, the blood sample collected, and then the remaining aspirated blood returned to the patient.

Table 4.4. Obtaining a Blood Sample from Arterial Line

- Turn off alarm.
- Remove cap from port closest to patient and maintain sterility.
- Attach a 10 ml syringe to the port closest to the patient. Turn stopcock "off" to transducer.
- Aspirate 3-5 ml of blood into syringe to clear the line of all intravenous fluids.
- Turn stopcock to halfway position so that it is "off" to transducer and patient.
- Remove syringe and discard.
- Attach sterile syringe to stopcock and turn stopcock "off" to transducer.
- Withdraw blood sample.
- Turn stopcock "off" to syringe port and "on" between patient and flush system.
- Remove the syringe.
- Flush the line.
- Turn the stopcock "off" to patient and "on" between flush system and port site.
- Flush the port site maintaining sterility of port.
- Put sterile cap on port.
- Re-establish the flush system and re-establish monitor alarms.

Removal of Arterial Line

In most critical care units, the RN discontinues the arterial line. See **Table 4.5** for an outline of the procedure.

Table 4.5. Removal of Arterial Line

- Close stopcock to patient and open transducer to air.
- Disconnect transducer from monitor, turn off alarms.
- Remove dressings and arterial catheter.
- Apply pressure with sterile gauze for 5 minutes or until bleeding stops.
- Apply a sterile pressure dressing to the site in accordance with hospital policy.
- Observe site for continued bleeding, normal circulation and sensation.

Selected References

Berne, Robert M., Levy, and Matthew N. *Cardiovascular Physiology.* (6th edition) Saint Louis: Mosby-Year Book, 1992.

Canobbio, Mary M. *Cardiovascular Disorders: Clinical Nursing Series.* Saint Louis: Mosby-Year Book, 1990.

Cheitlin, M., Sokolow, Maurice, and McIlroy, Malcolm. *Clinical Cardiology.* (6th edition) Connecticut: Appelton & Lange, 1993.

Civetta, J., Taylor, R., and Kirby. *Critical Care.* (2nd edition) Philadelphia: J.B. Lippincott Company, 1992.

Daily Elaine, and Schroeder, John. *Hemodynamic Waveforms.* (2nd edition) Saint Louis: The C.V. Mosby Company, 1990.

Daily, Elaine, and Schroeder, John. *Techniques in Bedside Hemodynamic Monitoring.* (5th edition) Saint Louis: The C.V. Mosby Company, 1994.

Gould, Kathleen Ahern. *Critical Care Nursing Clinics of North America,* Vol 1 (3), September 1989.

Guyton, Arthur C. *Textbook of Medical Physiology.* (8th edition) Philadelphia: W.B. Saunders Company, 1990.

Hand, Helen. "Direct or indirect blood pressure measurement. " *Critical Care Nurse,* 12(6), 52-59, 1992.

Henneman, Elizabeth, and Henneman, Philip. "Intricacies of blood pressure measurement: Reexamining the rituals." *Heart & Lung,* 18(3), 263-273, 1989.

Hudak, C., Gallo. *Critical Care Nursing: A Holistic Approach.* (6th edition) Philadelphia: J.B. Lippincott Company, 1994.

Katz, Arnold. *Physiology of the Heart.* (2nd edition) New York: Raven Press, 1992.

Kaye, William. "Invasive monitoring techniques: Arterial cannulation, bedside pulmonary artery catheterization, and arterial puncture."*Heart & Lung:* 12(4), 395-427, 1989.

Osguthorpe, Susan (Editor). "Physiologic monitoring." *AACN Clinical Issues in Critical Care Nursing.* 4(1), 1993.

CHAPTER FIVE

BASIC SKILLS IN ATRIAL PRESSURE MONITORING

Atrial pressure monitoring consists of right atrial pressure (RAP) or central venous pressure (CVP) monitoring and left atrial pressure (LAP) monitoring. The terms CVP and RAP will be used interchangeably in this chapter.

Indications for Invasive Central Venous Pressure Monitoring

- To continuously monitor the patient's blood volume or fluid status. It is most valuable in patients with active bleeding, recent surgery, or acute trauma.
- To obtain information regarding right ventricular (RV) function.

Insertion Sites

1. A central or peripheral vein may be used to insert a CVP catheter, and is accessed percutaneously or by venous cutdown.

2. The CVP catheter is inserted into the heart and positioned at the level of the superior vena cava or the mid-right atrium (See **Figure 5.1**). CXR should be done to confirm position.

3. Insertion sites include the internal and external jugular, subclavian, cephalic, femoral, and basilic veins.

4. The internal jugular and the subclavian veins are the most common sites of insertion.

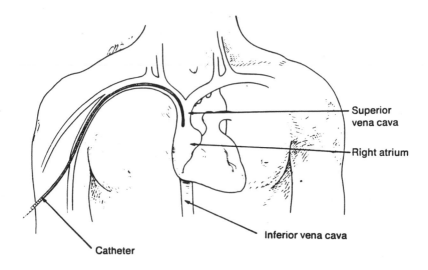

Figure 5.1. Position of CVP catheter. L.F. Abels. *Mosby's Manual of Critical Care.* Saint Louis: Mosby-Year Book, 1986. Used with permission of the publisher.

CVP Monitoring Equipment

1. CVP can be measured in centimeters of water (cm H2O) using a precalibrated manometer or in millimeters of mercury (mm Hg) using a pressure transducer system (Refer to **Table 5.1** for normal values).

Table 5.1. Normal CVP Values and Equation For Conversion

2-6 mm Hg or 3-8 cm H2O

To convert a reading from one form to another, the following equation may be utilized, since the two measurements are not interchangeable:

$$\frac{CVP \text{ in cm } H_2O}{1.36} = CVP \text{ in mm Hg}$$

2. Measuring CVP using a pressure transducer system is the most common method. The transducer converts pressure waves to electrical energy, which then can be displayed on an oscilloscope. The components of this system are the same as other invasive lines. Refer to Chapter 3 for a complete description of the equipment, calibration and zeroing techniques. **Table 5.2** describes the steps involved for measurement.

Table 5.2. Measuring CVP Using a Calibrated Transducer

- Wash hands.
- Calibrate and zero as outlined in Chapter 3.
- Place patient flat (or slightly elevated, NOT > 20˚) in supine position.
- Fast flush catheter if IV solution is not infusing.
- If IV fluid is running, turn stopcock at the transducer off to the intravenous fluid. The venous pressure waveform will now be visible on the oscilloscope.
- Observe the CVP tracing and note the respiratory cycles. The CVP reading should be taken at the same end-expiration period of two cycles.
- Return the stopcock to its normal position so that IV patency resumes if necessary.
- Wash hands and document in patient record.

3. CVP can also be measured with a plastic or glass precalibrated manometer. This technique is relatively simple and remains useful in the critical-care setting. The procedure is depicted in **Figure 5.2** and involves the steps described in **Table 5.3**.

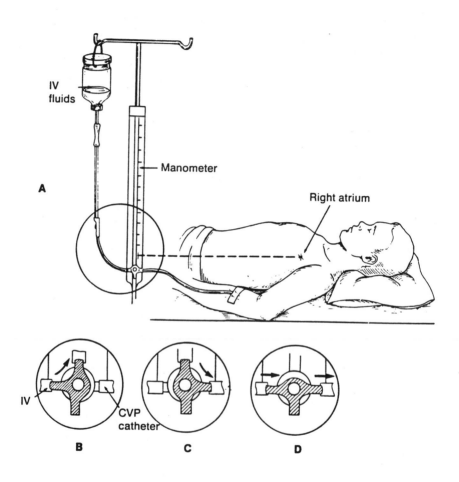

Figure 5.2. Procedure for CVP measurement utilizing a calibrated water manometer. A, Manometer and intravenous catheter in place. B, Stopcock turned to allow manometer to fill with fluid. C, Stopcock turned off to intravenous fluid to permit CVP reading. D, Stopcock in normal position, permitting resumption of intravenous flow to patient. L.F. Abels, *Mosby's Manual of Critical Care*. Saint Louis: Mosby-Year Book, 1986. Used by permission of the publisher.

Table 5.3. Calibrated Transducer Method

♦ Wash hands.

♦ Place patient flat (or slightly elevated, not > 20°) in supine position.

♦ The zero level of the manometer must be at the level of phlebostatic axis or the right atrium (mark point on chest so that future readings are taken at the same place).

♦ IV tubing is connected to a three-way stopcock at the base of the manometer, maintaining a closed system.

♦ Open IV tubing roller clamp and fill the manometer two-thirds full, clearing it completely of air bubbles.

♦ Turn stopcock to open manometer to patient and closed to the IV solution.

♦ Watch the fluid column fall quickly and then fluctuate at the point where the fluid column equalizes with the RA pressure (Fluid column will no longer drop.) The highest point of fluctuation is the CVP reading (end-expiration reading).

♦ Turn the stopcock off to manometer and resume IV flow (may need to adjust rate with roller clamp).

♦ Wash hands and document reading in centimeters of water pressure in the patient's record.

4. Respiratory variation must be taken into consideration when monitoring CVP. Any situation that alters intrathoracic pressure, such as spontaneous inspiration and mechanical ventilation, will affect the CVP waveform. For this reason, the CVP measurement should be read at the end of expiration for the most accurate information.

Pressure Wave Physiology and Contour

1. Central venous pressure (CVP) directly reflects right atrial pressure (RAP). Changes in CVP and potential etiologies for these are listed in **Table 5.4.**

Table 5.4. Etiologies for Changes in CVP

Conditions Causing Increased CVP

♦ Elevated intravascular volume

♦ High cardiac output (hyperdynamic cardiac function)

♦ Cardiac tamponade

♦ Pulmonary hypertension

♦ Vasopressor administration

♦ Depressed cardiac function (RV infarct, RV failure)

♦ Constrictive pericarditis

♦ Chronic left ventricular failure

Conditions Causing Decreased CVP

- Reduced intravascular volume
- Decreased mean systemic pressures (eg., as in early shock states)
- Venodilation (drug induced)

---

2. It indirectly reflects right ventricular preload or right ventricular end-diastolic pressure (RVEDP), as the tricuspid valve is open during diastole causing the right atrium and ventricle to become a common chamber.

3. It is influenced by the amount of blood in the right ventricle just before systole (preload), ventricular contractility, and the amount of resistance against which the right ventricle must eject blood (afterload).

4. In conditions where there is poor contractility, the right ventricle will not be able to empty completely, causing a rise in the right ventricular end diastolic pressure, and subsequently a rise in the CVP.

5. In conditions where there is increased afterload, such as from constriction of the pulmonary vessels or from obstruction to blood flow, i.e. pulmonary embolus, the CVP may rise.

6. Right atrial waveforms correspond to various phases in the cardiac cycle and consist of several deflections (See **Figure 5.3**).

   a. The "a" wave represents contraction of the right atrium (RA), or RA systole. It corresponds to PR interval on ECG (80 to 100 milliseconds after the P wave).

   b. The "c" wave, when seen, represents the tricuspid valve pushing into the right atrium as valve leaflets close during ventricular contraction (RST interval on ECG). It may appear as a distinct wave, as a notch on the "a" wave, or may be absent.

   c. The "v" wave represents passive atrial filling which occurs during ventricular systole as the right atrium fills with blood (latter half of the T wave on ECG).

   d. The "x" descent marks atrial diastole when there is a decrease in right atrial volume following atrial systole.

   e. The "y" descent immediately follows the "v" wave and represents emptying of the RA into the RV.

7. Recorded CVP waveforms lag slightly behind the corresponding ECG segment because the signal must travel through the long catheter before reaching the monitor. **Figure 5.4** depicts the right atrial pressure with the mechanical events (A and V waves) corresponding to the electrical events of the ECG.

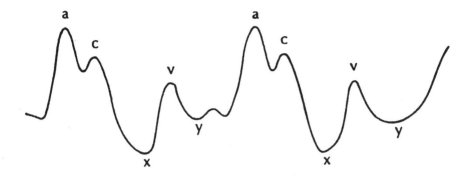

Figure 5.3 Right atrial pressure waveform. Seidel, Ball, Dains, Benedict, *Mosby's Guide to Physical Examination.* **(2nd edition) Saint Louis: Mosby-Year Book, 1991. From Malasangus, et. al., 1990. Used with permission of the publisher.**

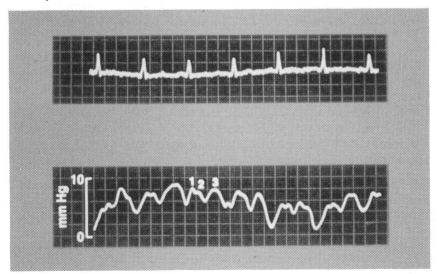

Key: 1= "a" wave
      2 = "c" wave
      3= "v" wave

Figure 5.4. Waveforms representing atrial and ventricular mechanical events followed by atrial and ventricular electrical events. Photos courtesy of Baxter Healthcare Corporation, Edwards-Critical Care Division. Used with permission.

8. RA pressures are recorded as a mean since there is only a very small pressure gradient between the high and low excursions of this waveform.

Caring for Patients with CVP Lines

Site

1. Cover with appropriate sterile dressing or immobilize site of insertion as needed.

2. Track date of insertion. Adhere to Center for Disease Control guidelines and hospital policy for how long catheter is to remain in place.

3. Change central line dressing in accordance with hospital policy, and observe site for signs of infection.

Equipment

1. Observe waveforms periodically on oscilloscope if the patient is being monitored with a transducer.

2. Troubleshoot any problems with waveforms and intervene as necessary (Refer to Monitoring Problems in Chapter 3).

3. Pressure tubing should be changed according to hospital policy.

4. CVP lines may be used for monitoring purposes, to infuse medications, or to obtain blood samples.

Complications

Complications associated with CVP catheters include pneumothorax, infection, and fluid overload (See **Table 5.5** for further description).

Table 5.5. Complications Associated with CVP Catheters

- **Pneumothorax**—may occur during insertion of the CVP line into the subclavian or jugular vein. Since the apex of the lung is in close proximity to these veins, it may be punctured accidently during insertion. A CXR must be taken after insertion of a CVP line to rule out its occurrence. This should be done prior to the infusion of other than KVO fluids (Normal Saline).

- **Infection**—may occur as the result of poor technique during insertion or dressing changes. Site must be observed for signs of infection including redness, swelling, warmth, or drainage. Temperature elevations should be noted.

- **Fluid overload**—to prevent accidental fluid overload, a controller or pump should be utilized to deliver prescribed IV fluids. Kinking of the tubing can occur, especially with jugular insertion sites. Jugular lines may be positional as the patient turns his/her head.

Indications for Invasive Left Atrial Pressure (LAP) Monitoring

1. To evaluate changes in cardiovascular hemodynamics that affect cardiac output following open heart surgery.

2. To obtain information regarding LV pressures.

3. To monitor patients with abnormal heart anatomy or other instances when a PA catheter is contraindicated.

4. To obtain information when PCWP pressure readings may be inaccurate, as in patients with high PAP's, or in the concomitant use of vasoconstricting medications and pulmonary vasodilator medications.

Insertion Site and Technique

1. A polyvinyl catheter (approximately 6 inches in length) is placed in the left atrium during open heart surgery.

2. Most common technique of insertion is through a needle puncture of the right superior pulmonary vein with subsequent threading into the left atrium.

3. Another method of insertion is via needle puncture directly into the left atrium at the intra-atrial groove just above the mitral valve.

4. The catheter is brought out through the chest wall (usually near the inferior portion of sternal incision).

LAP Monitoring Equipment

- LAP is recorded as a mean, and the normal range is 4 to 12 mm Hg.
- LAP line is connected to a pressure transducer system, and a continuous waveform is displayed on the oscilloscope. Refer to Chapter 3 for a complete description of the equipment, calibration and zeroing techniques. **Table 5.6** describes the steps involved for measurement.

Table 5.6. Obtaining LAP Measurement Utilizing a Calibrated Transducer

- ◆ Wash hands.
- ◆ Calibrate and zero as outlined in Chapter 3.
- ◆ Place patient flat (or slightly elevated, not> 20°) in supine position.
- ◆ Observe the LAP tracing and note the respiratory cycles. The LAP reading should be taken at the same end-expiration period of two cycles.
- ◆ Wash hands and document in patient's record.

Pressure Wave Physiology and Contour

1. Left atrial pressure (LAP) is a measurement of the pressure of blood as it returns to the left side of the heart. Changes in LAP and potential etiologies for these are listed in **Table 5.7.**

Table 5.7. Etiologies for Changes in LAP

Decreased LAP	Increased LAP
Fluid volume deficit	Fluid volume overload
	Impaired myocardial contractility
	Increased afterload
	Dysrhythmias
	Cardiac tamponade

2. It indirectly reflects left ventricular preload, as the mitral valve is opened during diastole causing the left atrium and ventricle to become a common chamber.

3. LAP provides the same information as the PCWP under most circumstances. Refer to Chapter 6 for review of PCWP.

4. Left atrial waveforms consist of several deflections and are similar in configuration to PCWP tracings.

   a. The "a" results from atrial contraction.

   b. The "c" wave reflects closure of the mitral valve.

   c. The "v" wave reflects atrial filling while the mitral valve is closed.

   d. The "x" descent marks atrial diastole or relaxation.

   e. The "y" descent immediately follows the "v" wave and represents emptying of the LA into the LV.

Caring for Patients with LA Lines

Site

1. Sterile dressing is placed over catheter exit site.

2. Track date of insertion. LAP catheter is normally used for 24-72 hours and then removed by a physician.

3. Change dressing in accordance with hospital policy (usually daily), and observe site for signs of infection.

Equipment

1. Observe waveforms periodically on oscilloscope.

2. Troubleshoot any unusual waveforms which may indicate catheter migration or air/clot in system (i.e. dampened wave form indicates air/clot in system and should not be used for readings until corrected; absent waveform may mean a clotted catheter or LV perforation).

3. Pressure tubing should be changed according to hospital policy.

4. LA Lines are to be used for pressure monitoring purposes only. **Do Not** use LA lines for infusion of medications, IV fluids or for blood samples. **Do Not** flush or irrigate LA lines.

Complications

1. Potential for air or blood clot emboli to enter the left atrium.

2. Potential for cardiac tamponade following LA line removal. This may occur if the small hole in the LA tissue does not clot and self-seal. If this does not occur, the patient will bleed into the pericardial space and develop tamponade.

Selected References

Boggs, R.L. and Wooldridge-King, M. (Editors) *AACN Procedure Manual For Critical Care*. (3rd edition) Philadelphia: W.B. Saunders Company, 1993.

Hartshorn, J., Lamborn, M., and Noll, M.L. *Introduction to Critical Care Nursing*. Philadelphia: W.B. Saunders Company, 1993.

Hudak, C.M., and Gallo, B.M. *Critical Care Nursing: A Holistic Approach*. Philadelphia: J.B. Lippincott Company, 1994.

Osguthorpe, S. (Guest Editor). *AACN Clinical Issues in Critical Care Nursing. Physiologic Monitoring*. Philadelphia: J.B. Lippincott Company, 1993.

Underhill, S.L., Woods, S.L., Froelicher, E.S., and Halpenny, C.J. *Cardiac Nursing* (2nd edition) Philadelphia: J.B. Lippincott Company, 1989.

Wilson, R.B. *Critical Care Manual: Applied Physiology and Principles of Therapy*. (2nd edition) Philadelphia: F.A. Davis Company, 1992.

Wright, J.E. and Shelton, B.K. *Desk Reference for Critical Care Nursing*. Boston: Jones and Bartlett Publishers, 1993.

CHAPTER SIX

UNRAVELLING PULMONARY ARTERY PRESSURE MONITORING

The pulmonary artery catheter is a balloon-tipped, flow directed catheter that is placed in the pulmonary artery, then attached to a high pressure, fluid filled system allowing for continuous pressure monitoring.

Indications for Pulmonary Artery Pressure Monitoring

- To measure the right atrial (RA), right ventricular (RV), pulmonary artery (PA), pulmonary capillary wedge (PCW) pressures of the heart.
- To assess the fluid status of the patient.
- To monitor the cardiac output.
- To evaluate the oxygen supply and demand.
- To differentiate noncardiac from cardiac pulmonary edema.
- To diagnose and differentiate various cardiac diseases.

In summary, the pulmonary artery catheter allows the clinician to evaluate the hemodynamic status of the patient and the effectiveness of therapies.

Components of a Pulmonary Artery Catheter

The catheter consists of a right atrial port or proximal port, a right ventricular pacing port, and a pulmonary artery port or distal port. In addition, it has a balloon inflation port and a connection for the thermistor for cardiac output. Sometimes there are two proximal ports and a pulmonary artery port in place of the right ventricular pacing port. (**Figure 6.1**)

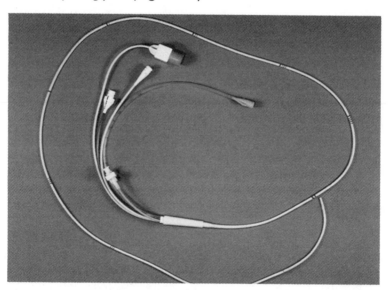

Figure 6.1. Pulmonary artery catheter

1. The **RA (right atrial) port** is located in the right atrium. It can be connected to a high-pressure, fluid-filled tubing for continuous or intermittent right atrial or CVP readings. This port is also the injectate port for the cardiac output. If there is a second right atrial port, it is used for fluid infusion.

2. The **RV (right ventricular) pacing port** is located in the right ventricle. It is utilized for placement of a right ventricular pacing wire and/or fluid infusion.

3. The **PA (pulmonary artery) port** is located in the pulmonary artery and is **always** connected to a high-pressure, fluid-filled tubing for a continuous display of the PA pressure.

4. The **balloon inflation port** allows for instillation of air into the balloon at the catheter tip for temporary wedging and display of the pulmonary capillary wedge pressure.

5. The **thermistor** is a temperature monitoring device that connects to a computer which measures and displays the cardiac output. For more information about the monitoring system and pressure tubing refer to Chapter Three.

Insertion

The pulmonary artery (PA) catheter is inserted into the pulmonary artery via one of the following vessels:
- Subclavian vein
- Internal jugular vein
- External jugular vein
- Femoral vein
- Antecubital vein (via cutdown)

Setup

Prior to insertion:

1. Assemble all necessary equipment. This varies from institution to institution.

2. Flush each port of the PA catheter with normal saline. The distal port is flushed with the heparinized solution from the fluid-filled pressure tubing.

3. Maintaining sterility, wipe the exterior of the PA catheter with a sterile solution.

4. Check the integrity of the balloon by inflating with 1.5 cc of air. (Note: check the shaft of the catheter for the recommended amount of air.)

5. Position the patient according to the access to be utilized, as well as the patient's tolerance.

6. Balance and calibrate the transducer. The transducer air-fluid interface should be placed at the phlebostatic axis. For further details refer to Chapter Three.

Cannulation

This procedure is done under strict aseptic technique. The person inserting the catheter should wear a sterile gown and gloves in addition to a cap and protective eye wear.

1. The vessel to be cannulated will be selected by the physician. The antecubital vein needs to be accessed by cutdown. All other vessels mentioned above can be cannulated percutaneously.

2. The site for insertion is prepped with a betadine solution; then the patient is draped accordingly. The insertion site should be injected with a local anesthetic for patient comfort.

3. Once the vessel is accessed, a guidewire is placed through the introducer needle and the needle is removed. The catheter introducer is placed over the guidewire and the guidewire is removed.

Insertion of the Pulmonary Artery Catheter

Nursing Responsibilities

1. Explain the procedure to the patient.

2. Monitor the patient's cardiac rhythm throughout the procedure as ventricular arrhythmias may occur upon insertion of the catheter.

3. Have emergency medications available, in particular lidocaine for ventricular arrhythmias.

4. Have a defibrillator available for ventricular arrhythmias.

5. Monitor all other vital signs, in particular the respiratory rate and depth as some patients cannot tolerate lying flat for any period of time.

6. Run a continuous strip of pressure tracings during insertion.

7. Document and record all pressures throughout insertion.(Refer to **figures 6.1A, 6.1B, 6.1C**)

8. Provide reassurance throughout the procedure.

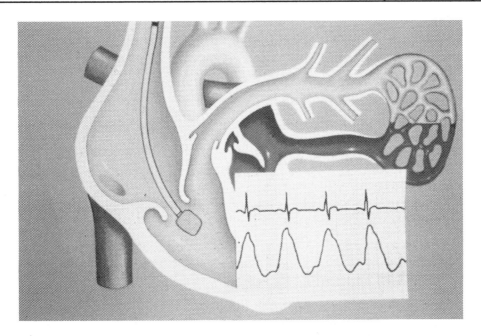

Figure 6.1A-Pulmonary Artery Catheter insertion- Right Ventricle. Photos courtesy of Baxter Healthcare Corporation, Edwards- Critical Care Division. Used with permission. Photos couresy of Baxter Healthcare Corporation,, Edwards-Critical Care Division. Used with permission

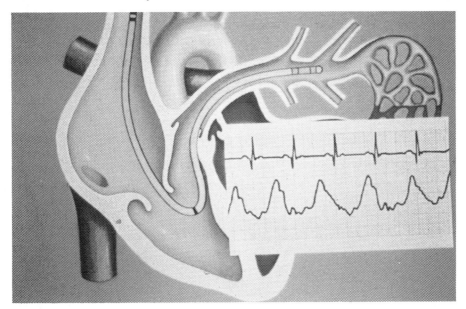

Figure 6.1B- Pulmonary Artery Catheter insertion-Pulmonary Artery. Photos courtesy of Baxter Healthcare Corporation, Edwards-Critical care Division. Used with permission.

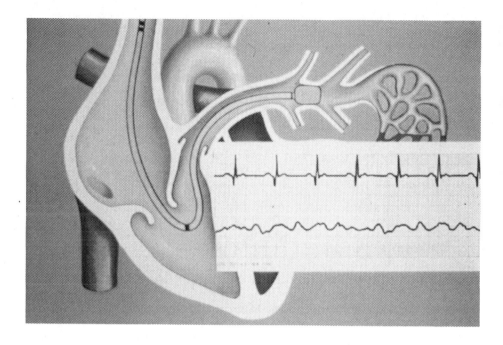

Figure 6.1C- Pulmonary Artery Catheter insertion- Wedge Position. Photos courtesy of Baxter Healthcare Corporation, Edwards-Critical Care Divivision. Used with permission.

Physician Responsibilities

1. Obtain informed consent.

2. Wash hands and don mask, cap, eye wear, and sterile gown and gloves.

3. Prep the site and drape the patient.

4. Inject a local anesthetic.

5. Prepare the catheter as stated above under "setup". Make certain all lumens are flushed and the distal port (PA port) is connected to the pressure line. Cover the PA catheter with the protective sheath. This sheath allows for repositioning of the catheter without the risk of contamination. (**Figure 6.2**)

6. Once the vessel is cannulated and the introducer guidewire is in place, thread the PA catheter through the catheter introducer. (**Figure 6.3 and 6.4**)

7. When the catheter is in the superior vena cava, partially inflate the balloon. The inflation of the balloon will assist the passage of the catheter into the right atrium. Once in the right atrium, inflate the balloon with about 1 cc to assist with floating the catheter into the right ventricle and then into the pulmonary artery.

   Position of the catheter is monitored by the waveform displayed. The waveform displayed is what is seen by the distal tip of the PA catheter. This waveform in addition to the cardiac monitor must be monitored throughout insertion.

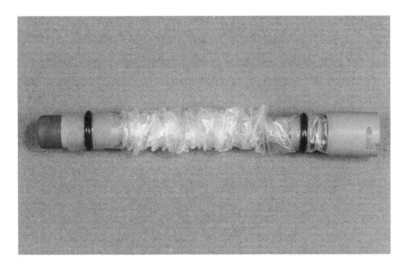

Figure 6.2. Sheath for pulmonary artery catheter

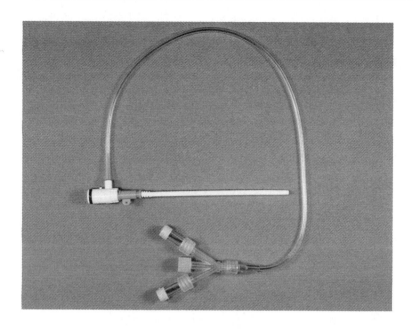

Figure 6.3. Introducer for pulmonary artery catheter.

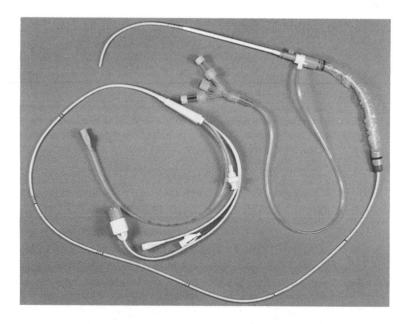

Figure 6.4. Pulmonary artery catheter with sheath in place through introducer.

8. Once in place, suture the catheter introducer in place and apply a sterile dressing. Confirm position of the catheter by chest X-ray.

Waveform Analysis

Right Atrial Pressure Waveform

The right atrial waveform consists of three positive deflections, the a wave, c wave and v wave respectively. (**Figure 6.5**)

Right Atrial Waveform

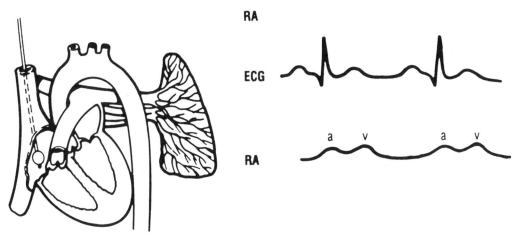

Figure 6.5. Right atrial pressure waveform with corresponding ECG. Photos courtesy of Baxter Healthcare Corporation, Edwards-Critical Care Division. Used with permission.

1. **A WAVE:** reflects pressure during right atrial contraction. It can be seen right after the p wave on the ECG. (Refer to **Figure 6.5**)

2. **C WAVE:** reflects pressure during tricuspid valve closure. It can be seen after the QRS complex on the ECG. It is not always visible.

3. **V WAVE:** reflects peak RA pressure just prior to tricuspid valve opening. It can be seen during the latter half of the T wave on the ECG. (Refer to **Figure 6.5**)

Measurement of RA Pressures

Pressures are measured as a mean. Because there is not a great difference between the pressures during atrial systole (a wave) and atrial diastole (v wave), a mean of all the waves is taken. When there is a difference between the a wave and v wave greater than 3-4 mm Hg, the mean of the a wave should be taken. Normal pressures are from 2 mm Hg-6 mm Hg.

RA pressures can also be measured in cm of water using a water manometer. The use of disposable transducers has caused limited use of water manometers. Because use of water manometers in non-critical care units is still common, an understanding of the relationship between water measurement and Hg measurement is necessary. The relationship between cm of water and mm of Hg is not 1:1, however. Hg is heavier than water. Centimeters of water can be converted to mm of Hg by dividing centimeters of water by 1.36. Another method of conversion is to multiply cm of water by 0.74 mm of Hg.

$$6 \text{ cm } H_2O = \frac{6 \text{ cm } H_2O}{1.36} = 4.4 \text{ mm Hg}$$

or

$$6 \text{ cm } H_2O = 6 \text{ cm } H_2O \times 0.74 \text{ mm Hg} = 4.4 \text{ mm Hg}$$

Right Ventricular Pressure Waveform

The pressure waveforms seen when the PA catheter enters the right ventricle reflects systole and diastole of the right ventricle. (**Figure 6.6**)

Right Ventricular Waveform

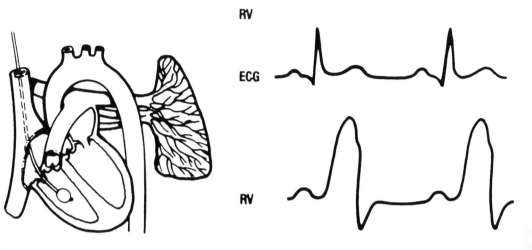

Figure 6.6. Right venticular pressure waveform with corresponding ECG. Photos courtesy of Baxter Healthcare Corporation, Edwards-Critical Care Division. Used with permission.

1. The systolic pressure waveforms generated in the right ventricle reflect the two phases of this cycle, isovolumetric contraction and ejection. (For further explanation refer to Chapter One, cardiac cycle. The reflective wave shows rapid filling, a slow filling and an a wave which represents atrial systole.

2. Systole can be seen during the QT interval of the ECG **(Figure 6.6)**. Normal systolic pressure ranges from 15-28 mm Hg.

3. The diastolic pressure waveforms generated in the right ventricle reflect the four phases of this cycle, isovolumetric relaxation, rapid filling of the ventricle, slow filling of the ventricle, and atrial systole. (For further explanation refer to Chapter One, cardiac cycle.)

4. Diastole can be seen between the TQ interval of the ECG (Refer to **Figure 6.6**). Normal diastolic pressure ranges from 2-6 mm Hg. Because the tricuspid valve is open during diastole, the pressures in the right atrium and right ventricle should be the same.

(Note: the right ventricular pressure is not routinely monitored continuously. It is usually monitored only during insertion.)

Pulmonary Artery Pressure Waveform

1. The pressure waveform seen when the PA catheter enters the pulmonary artery reflects systolic and diastolic pressure in the pulmonary artery. **(Figure 6.7)**

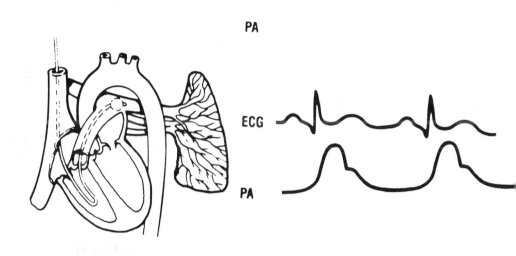

Figure 6.7. Pulmonary artery pressure waveform with corresponding ECG. Courtesy of Baxter Healthcare Corporation, Edwards-Critical Care Division. Used with permission.

2. During systole, the pulmonic valve opens allowing for rapid flow of blood from the right ventricle. Since there is an open channel between the right ventricle and the pulmonary artery at this time, the pressure in the pulmonary artery and the right ventricle during systole should be the same (15-28 mm Hg). This waveform should correspond with the QT interval on the ECG. (Refer to **Figure 6.7.**)

3. The beginning of diastole follows the closure of the pulmonic valve. This is reflected as a notch on the waveform called the dicrotic notch. The end diastolic pressure corresponds with the left ventricular end diastolic pressure because there are no valves between the pulmonary artery, pulmonary vasculature, left atrium, and left ventricle, with the exception of the mitral valve which is open during diastole. Normal PA diastolic pressure is 8 mm Hg-16 mm Hg.

Note: Although normal pressures are listed in this text, there are reasons why the patient may have pressures that are out of these ranges and they will still be normal.

Pulmonary Capillary Wedge Pressure

When the balloon port of the pulmonary artery catheter is inflated, the catheter should float into a small branch of the pulmonary artery, occluding flow to that portion of the pulmonary artery. This prevents flow from the right side of the heart to that vessel. Pressure in that vessel is reflective of pressure in the left atrium again because there are no valves between the catheter tip and the left atrium (**Figure 6.8**).

Figure 6.8. Pulmonary capillary wedge pressure waveform with corresponding ECG. Courtesy of Baxter Healthcare Corporation, Edwards-Critical Care Division. Used with permission.

Pulmonary Artery Wedge Waveform

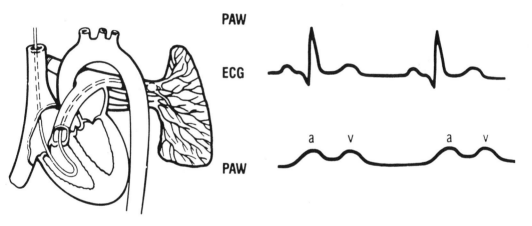

1. The pressure waveform is similar to that of the pressure wave form of the right atrium.

    •   **A WAVE:** reflects pressure during left atrial contraction. This can be seen after the p wave on the ECG.

    •   **C WAVE :** reflects pressure from the closure of the mitral valve. This is not normally visible.

    •   **V WAVE :** reflects pressure during filling of the left atrium and the bulging back of the mitral valve during ventricular systole. This can be seen following the T wave on the ECG. (**Figure 6.8**)

2. The presence of these waves in both the right atrium and left atrium are dependant upon normal electrical conduction. If there are no p waves, there will be no a waves.

3. Measurement of the pulmonary artery wedge pressure is a mean pressure of the a and v waves. Normal pulmonary capillary wedge pressure (PCWP) is 6 mm Hg-12 mm Hg.

4. The pulmonary capillary wedge pressure in individuals with no preexisting pulmonary problems is close to that of the pulmonary artery diastolic pressure (PAD). In fact the PCWP is slightly lower than that of the PAD. It must be, in order to allow for forward flow of blood. If a pulmonary capillary wedge pressure reading is higher than that of the pulmonary artery diastolic reading, there must be an error in the reading.

Measurement of Pulmonary Artery Pressures

All pulmonary artery pressures, systolic , diastolic, and wedge, should be taken at end-expiration. The reason for this is that at end expiration there is the least variance in intrathoracic pressure.

1. When a patient is breathing spontaneously, the pressure in the pulmonary artery is elevated upon expiration. The reading should be taken just prior to the fall in pressure.

2. When a patient is on mechanical ventilation, the pressure in the pulmonary artery rises upon inspiration and falls during expiration. The reading should be taken just prior to the rise in pressure (**Figure 6.9**).

3. Those patients who are on intermittent mandatory ventilation will have some spontaneous breaths and some ventilator breaths. In this case, readings should be taken from graphic recordings, or by observing the patient's breathing and measuring accordingly.

4. If the patient is on PEEP, the clinician should NOT remove the patient from the ventilator to obtain pressure readings.

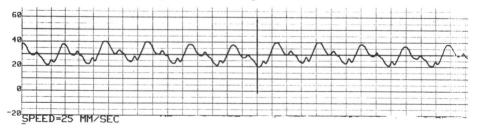

Figure 6.9. Measurement of the PAD on mechanical ventilation. Measurement of the PA diastolic should be taken at end expiration designated by the line in the above figure. Inspiration in the mechanically ventilated patient occurs after the line.

Table 6.1 Causes of High and Low Pressure Readings

READING	HIGH READINGS	LOW READINGS
RA	RV failure Tricuspid stenosis/ insufficiency Tamponade Pulmonary embolus Pulmonary HTN Obstructive pulmonary disease Chronic LV failure Volume overload	Hypovolemia Sepsis Cirrhosis Anemia Beri-Beri
RV DIAS	RV failure Tricuspid stenosis / insufficiency Tamponade Pulmonary embolus Pulmonary HTN Obstructive pulmonary disease Chronic LV failure Volume overload	Hypovolemia Sepsis Cirrhosis Beri-Beri

Note: RA and RVD causes for elevated pressure are the same due to the open tricuspid valve.

READING	HIGH READINGS	LOW READINGS
RV SYST	Pulmonary HTN	Hypovolemia
	Pulmonary embolus	Sepsis
	Hypoxemia	Cirrhosis
	ARDS	Anemia
	Obstructive lung disease	Beri-Beri
	VSD	
	Pulmonic stenosis	
	Left ventricular failure	
PA DIAS	Elevated pulmonary/ vascular resistance	Hypovolemia
		Sepsis
	Pulmonary embolus	Cirrhosis
	Tachycardia	Anemia
	Pulmonary disease	Beri-Beri
	ARDS	
	Left ventricular failure	
	Fluid overload	
PA SYST	Shunting (AV defects)	Hypovolemia
	Constrictive pericarditis	Sepsis
	Hypoxemia	Cirrhosis
	COPD	Anemia
	ARDS	Beri-Beri
	Left ventricular failure	
	Fluid overload	

READING	HIGH READINGS	LOW READINGS
PCWP	Left ventricular failure	Hypovolemia
	Fluid overload	Sepsis
	Mitral stenosis or insufficiency	Cirrhosis
		Anemia
	Tamponade	Beri-Beri
	Pericardial effusion	
	Decreased LV compliance	
	Positive pressure ventilation	

Table 6.2. Complications of Pulmonary Artery Catheters

PROBLEM	CAUSES	INTERVENTIONS
Waveform problems	See Chapter Four	See Chapter Four
Kinked catheter	Excessive length of catheter inserted (eg. severe dilation of RV)	Withdraw and reinsert
	Sharp angle of insertion	Reinsert, or reposition
Knotting	Excessive length of catheter inserted (eg. severe dilation of RV)	Under fluoroscopy remove the catheter
Dysrhythmia	Irritation of the endocardium	Inflate the balloon during insertion; limit time in the ventricle
	Direct injury to conduction bundles	Remove the catheter when no longer clinically necessary
	Damage to the tricuspid and pulmonic valves	Remove the catheter when no longer necessary

PROBLEM	CAUSES	INTERVENTIONS
Infection	Break in sterile technique upon insertion	Maintain sterile technique
	Contamination of the system during use, or calibration	Limit the number of times the system is interrupted
	Non-occlusive dressing	Apply an occlusive dressing
Balloon rupture	Frequent inflation	Limit balloon inflation
	Gradual loss of elasticity	Limit balloon inflation
	Overinflation	Use only amount of air necessary to produce a wedge waveform
Air embolus	Balloon rupture	Seal balloon if it has ruptured and have the catheter removed or replaced
	Improper technique in removing the catheter and introducer	Remove the catheter with the patient in the supine position and apply direct pressure over the insertion site upon withdrawal of the catheter
Pulmonary infarction/rupture	Overinflation of the balloon	Only inflate with the recommended amount of air, and only inflate until a wedge tracing appears
	Prolonged wedging	Inflate balloon for intermittent readings
	Vigorous flushing of the PA catheter	Avoid flushing of the distal port
	Thrombus formation at the end of the catheter	Keep catheter patent with continuous flush device
	Catheter migration	Monitor tip pressure continuously
	Pulmonary HTN	Identify patients at risk

PROBLEM	CAUSES	INTERVENTIONS
Wedge tracing	Catheter not in proper position	Have catheter repositioned
	Incorrect amount of air inserted	See above Check the shaft of the catheter for the correct amount of air to be instilled
Thrombocytopenia	Heparin flush solution	Remove the heparin from the flush solution

Obtaining the Pulmonary Artery Pressures

1. Explain the procedure to the patient.

2. With a carpenter's level, maintain the air-fluid interface at the level of the phlebostatic axis. This point should be marked on the patient for future readings. (See Chapter Four)

3. Open the transducer stopcock to air and off to the patient. Remove the dead-ender cap. Maintain sterility of the cap and the rest of the system.

4. Zero the system.

5. Calibrate the paper.

6. Run the strip recorder.

7. Turn the stopcock off to air and open to patient, replacing a sterile dead-ender cap.

8. Read the PA pressures at end expiration. (See previous section on measurement of pulmonary artery pressures.)

9. Wedge the catheter. (See procedure for obtaining wedge pressures.)

Obtaining Pulmonary Capillary Wedge Pressures

1. Explain the procedure to the patient.

2. Follow steps 2-7 above.

3. Draw the recommended volume of air into the balloon syringe.

4. Attach to the balloon port and open the port.

5. While observing the tracing on the monitor, slowly inject the air into the balloon port until a pulmonary capillary wedge tracing appears **(Figure 6.10)**. A small amount of resistance should be felt when inflating the balloon. The balloon should not remain inflated for greater than four respiratory cycles.

6. Read the PCWP at end expiration, taking a mean of the a and v waves.

7. Allow for passive deflation of the balloon by removing your finger from the plunger of the syringe. Then remove the syringe from the port.

8. Observe for return of the pulmonary artery tracing.

Note: If a wedge tracing appears at a volume of less than 1cc, notify the MD to pull the catheter back to a position where a wedge tracing is obtained with the full inflation volume.

Wedging Techniques

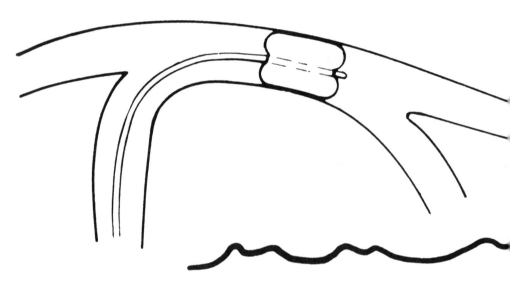

Proper Wedge

Figure 6.10. Courtesy of Baxter Healthcare Corporation, Edwards-Critical Care Division. Used with permission.

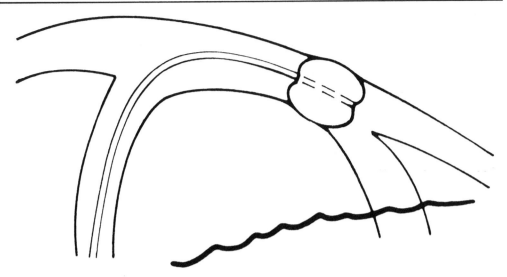

Overinflation

Figure 6.11. Courtesy of Baxter Healthcare Corporation. Edwards Critical-Care Division. Used with permission.

Obtaining a Blood Sample from the Pulmonary Artery Catheter for Mixed Venous Oxygen Saturation

1. Explain the procedure to the patient.

2. Wash hands.

3. Gather a 5 cc syringe, heparinized syringe, 10 cc syringe, and a 2 × 2 gauze pad.

4. Don non-sterile gloves.

5. Remove the dead-ender cap and attach a 5 cc syringe to the top port of the stopcock closest to the catheter distal port.

6. Turn stopcock off to the pressure tubing, and aspirate blood.

7. Turn stopcock off to the syringe and remove and discard the syringe in an appropriate receptacle. Attach the heparinized syringe to the stopcock and open the stopcock to the syringe.

8. Withdraw blood sample SLOWLY to prevent contamination of mixed venous blood with arterial blood from a capillary from the pulmonary artery.

9. Turn stopcock off to the syringe, remove syringe, label, and place on ice.

10. Place 10 cc syringe on stopcock and turn stopcock off to the patient. Fill the syringe with approximately 5 cc of the flush solution.

11. Turn stopcock off to the pressure tubing and open to the patient and aspirate until blood enters the syringe. Assure that no clots are visible. Flush the catheter with the flush solution from the syringe.

12. Turn the stopcock off to the syringe. Remove the syringe and discard in an appropriate receptacle.

13. Turn the stopcock off to the patient and open to air. Flush the top port of the stopcock with the flush solution into a 2 × 2 gauze pad.

14. Turn the stopcock off to the top port and replace the sterile dead-ender cap.

15. Ensure that the pressure tracing has returned to the oscilloscope.

16. Remove gloves, discard and wash hands.

Note: For more information on mixed venous oxygen monitoring see Chapter 7.

Cardiac Output Measurement

For a full explanation of cardiac output and the factors affecting cardiac output, refer to Chapter One "Cardiac Output and Factors Affecting Cardiac Output." To understand the technique of cardiac output measurement, a full understanding of the facts presented in Chapter One is essential.

1. Methods utilized to determine cardiac output include:

    - Fick method
    - Indicator dilution method
    - Thermodilution method
    - Thoracic electrical bioimpedence - not widely accepted or used
    - Noninvasive measurement of SV then calculate CO and CI

2. In critical care settings, cardiac output measurement is generally performed utilizing the thermodilution method.

3. For an explanation of the Fick and the indicator-dilution methods, refer to the references at the end of this chapter.

Thermodilution Cardiac Output Measurement

1. Cardiac output measurement utilizing this method requires installation of a known temperature solution, either iced or room temperature, through the proximal lumen of a pulmonary artery catheter. The change in temperature is detected by a thermistor which is located 4 cm from the catheter tip. This temperature change is displayed as a curve by the cardiac output computer. (**Figure 6.12**)

2. The thermodilution method can be accomplished utilizing a closed system or an open system. Both procedures will be described here.

3. There are several factors that must be observed before performing cardiac output determination:

   a. PA waveform must be assessed for correct placement to avoid errors in readings.

   b. Computation constant on the computer must be appropriate for the particular catheter, volume of injectate, iced or room temperature, and the computer being used.

4. Computation constant and the blood temperature in the pulmonary artery are incorporated into the equation by the computer to determine cardiac output.

5. The clinician must make certain that the computation constant is entered accurately prior to cardiac output measurement.

Cardiac Output Measurement Utilizing the Closed Injectate System

1. Explain the procedure to the patient.

2. Wash hands.

3. Gather all equipment; closed system for cardiac output (CO set), D_5W IV bag, cardiac output computer and cable.

4. Close clamp on CO set and spike IV bag.

5. Uncoil CO set to desired length and attach the 10 ml CO syringe.

6. Tighten all connections, then flush the system through by opening the clamp.

7. Slowly pull the plunger on the syringe to prime the system. Repeat the procedure until all air is flushed from the system.

8. Close the clamp and empty the syringe of all fluid.

9. Attach the CO set to a stopcock on the proximal injectate port on the PA catheter.

10. Attach temperature probe to the CO set.

11. Attach cardiac output computer cable to the PA catheter.

12. Enter the appropriate computation constant.

13. Observe the PA catheter waveform for correct placement.

14. Check for a ready indicator on the cardiac output computer.

15. Make certain the start button is within reach.

16. Open the clamp to the injectate solution and fill the syringe with 10 cc of fluid. 5cc of fluid may be used with patients who are fluid restricted.

17. Limit the amount of handling of the syringe as it may alter the temperature.

18. Observe the patient's respiratory pattern.

19. Upon end-expiration push the start button on the computer and begin injection of the syringe contents. Inject over a 4 second period, or inject 5cc in 2 seconds.

20. Observe the CO curve on the CO computer. It should have a smooth rapid upstroke indicating a rapid even injection, and an even downslope (**Figure 6.12**).

21. Repeat steps 13-20 for two more CO measurements. An average of the three measurements is taken providing there isn't greater than a 10% difference between them.

22. Record the measurement on the patient's record.

23. Return the stopcock so that the infusion/pressure recording continues.

NOTE: Continuous infusions, particularly vasopressors, should not be infused via the injectate port because performing cardiac outputs will cause the patient to be bolused with the medication.

Normal Cardiac Output

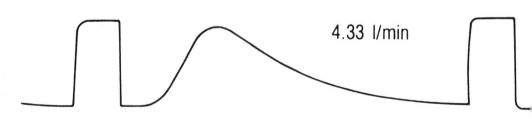

4.33 l/min

Figure 6.12 Normal cardiac output curve. Courtesy of Baxter Healthcare Corporation, Edwards-Critical Care Division. Used with permission.

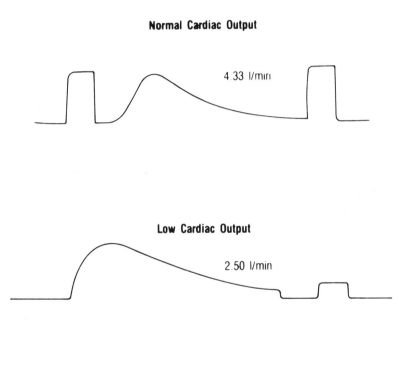

Normal Cardiac Output

4.33 l/min

Low Cardiac Output

2.50 l/min

High Cardiac Output

8.21 l/min

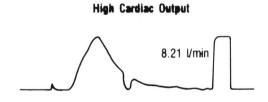

Figure 6.13. Comparison of normal, low, and high cardiac output. Courtesy of Baxter Healthcare Corporation, Edwards-Critical Care Division. Used with permission.

Closed Injectate Delivery System, Cold

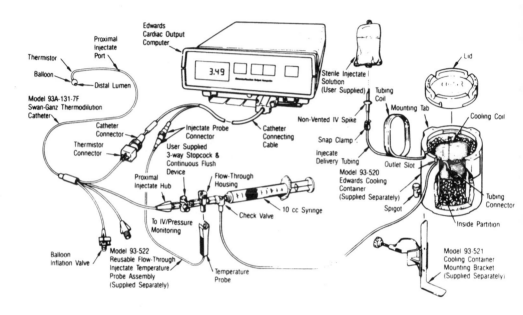

Figure 6.14. Courtesy of Baxter Healthcare Corporation, Edwards-Critical Care Divison. Used with permission.

Cardiac Output Measurement Utilizing the Open Injectate System

1. Explain the procedure to the patient.

2. Wash hands.

3. Gather equipment; D5W, (4) 10 cc syringes ,(4) 20 gauge needles, polyethylene bag, cardiac output computer, alcohol swabs.

4. Attach needles to syringes and withdraw 10 cc of D5W in each after swabbing the injection port with alcohol.

5. Remove the needles and replace with injection caps.

6. Place the syringes in the polyethylene bag and seal shut.

7. Attach the cardiac output computer to the PA catheter.

8. Enter in the appropriate computation constant.

9. Observe the PA waveform for correct placement of the catheter.

10. Open the polyethylene bag and remove the plunger from one syringe. Place the temperature probe in the syringe. Close the bag and place the bag in a container.

11. Do not handle the barrel of the syringes as this may alter the temperature.

12. Check to see if the CO computer is ready and the start button in reach.

13. Open the bag with the syringes and remove one. Attach to the stopcock on the proximal injectate (RA) port of the PA catheter.

14. The stopcock should be located between the catheter and the pressure (IV infusion) tubing.

15. Upon end-expiration, depress the start button and inject the contents of the syringe, smoothly and rapidly (over 4 sec).

16. Observe the curve for a rapid upstroke and a smooth return to baseline.

17. Repeat steps 12-16 two more times. An average of the three readings is taken provided there isn't greater than a 10% difference between them.

18. Return the stopcock to the upright position and replace the dead-ender cap.

Continuous Cardiac Output Measurement

Continuous cardiac output (CCO) measurement is available by utilizing a continuous cardiac output pulmonary artery catheter. This catheter insertion technique is the same as the pulmonary artery catheter.

Indications for Continuous Cardiac Output Monitoring

- To provide continuous monitoring of cardiac output in compromised contractility states.
- Evaluate therapeutic modalities—Inotropic drugs.
- Detect immediate changes in critically ill patients.

Advantages

- Provides continuous monitoring
- Decreases risk of fluid overload
- Decreases risk of infections
- Gives early indication of changes (e.g. cardiogenic shock)
- Decreases error in fluctuating boluses

Principles of Continuous Cardiac Output Monitoring

1. **Heated filament** is wrapped around pulmonary artery catheter at the injectate port.

2. Energy signals (heat) are infused from the injectate port into the blood in a continuous on/off pattern.

3. Heat signal is then sensed in the blood near the tip of the catheter.

4. "A microcomputer-based instrument samples the filament input sequence and the distal thermistors response to the blood warming"(Yeldman, 1993, p.129). This is indicative of the time it takes the warmed blood to travel from the entry site to the distal port.

5. This signal is calculated over a three-minute period of time and a curve is formed on the monitor.

6. The cardiac output (CO) is calculated from the area under the curve.

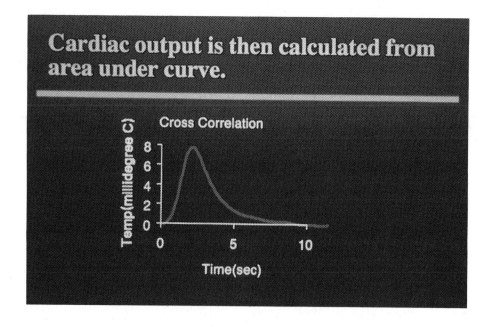

Figure 6.15 Photo courtesy of Baxter Healthcare Corporation, Edwards-Critical Care Division. Used with permission.

7. The cardiac output displayed is an average of the previous 3-6 minutes. This is referred to as "Time- Averaging" and represents a trend of CO. The display is updated every 30-60 minutes.

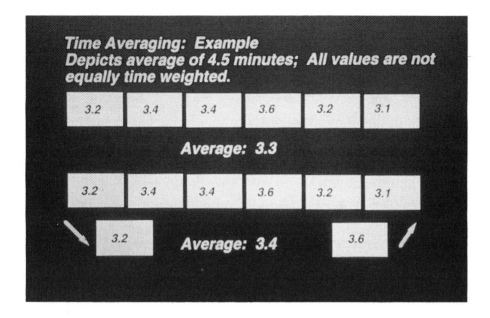

Figure 6.16. Photos courtesy of Baxter Healthcare Corporation, Edwards-Critical Care Division. Used with permission.

Troubleshooting Continuous Cardiac Output Monitoring

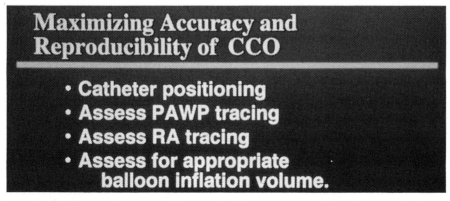

Figure 6.17. Photos courtesy of Baxter Healthcare Corporation, Edwards-Critical Care Division. Used with permission.

For additional troubleshooting of the CCO catheter, refer to **Table 6.3** on troubleshooting the cardiac output measurements.

Table 6.3 Troubleshooting Cardiac Output Measurements

PROBLEM	CAUSE	SOLUTION
Variation of >10%	Uneven injection	Inject smoothly over 4 sec
	Patient movement	Limit movement
	Room temperature injectate	Use iced injectate
	Dysrhythmia	Correct dysrhythmia
	Catheter whip	Reposition catheter
	Injection during different phases of the respiratory cycle	Inject during end expiration
Values too high	Too little injectate	Measure injectate carefully
	Temperature too warm	Check injectate temperature carefully
	Computation constant set too high	Check computation constant
	Uneven injection	Inject smoothly over 4 sec
Values too low	Too much injectate	Measure injectate carefully
	Injection of solution prior to depressing start	Depress start prior to injection
	Injectate too warm	Check injectate temperature prior to injection
	Computation constant set too low	Check computation constant
	Prolonged injection	Inject over 4 sec

Table 6.3 continued.

PROBLEM	CAUSE	SOLUTION
	Use of normal saline	Use D$_5$W
Unable to inject solution	Proximal port clotted	Notify physician
	Port kinked	Notify physician to reposition
	Stopcock in the off position	Check all stopcocks
Variation in core temperature	Faulty thermistor	Replace PA catheter
	Fibrin growth on thermistor	Replace PA catheter

Table 6.4. Non-Technical Causes For Alterations In Cardiac Output

Low Cardiac Output	– M.I.
	– Valvular heart disease
	– CHF
	– Tamponade
	– Myocarditis
	– Hypovolemia
	– Positive pressure ventilation
	– Cardiogenic shock
High Cardiac Output	– Septic shock
	– Thiamine deficiency
	– Thyrotoxicosis
	– Sympathetic stimulation
	– Anemia
	– Cirrhosis
	– Paget's disease

Selected References

Aherns, T., and Taylor, L. *Hemodynamic Wave Form Analysis*. Philadelphia: W.B.Saunders Company, 1992.

Baxter-Edwards. *Continuous Cardiac Output*. California: Baxter Healthcare Corporation, 1993.

Daily, Elaine,and Schroeder, John *Techniques in Bedside Hemodynamic Monitoring*. (4th edition) Saint Louis: The C.V. Mosby Company, 1989.

Dennison, R.D. "Making sense of hemodynamic monitoring." *AJN*, Aug., 24-32, 1994.

Gardner, Polly E. "Pulmonary artery pressure monitoring." *AACN Clinical Issues in Critical Care Nursing*, 4(1), 98-119, 1993.

Kern, L. "Hemodynamic monitoring." *AACN Procedure Manual for Critical Care*. (3rd edition) Philadelphia: W.B. Saunders Company, 1993.

McIntire, B. "Troubleshooting invasive hemodynamic monitoring systems." *Critical Care Choices*. 43-46, 1993.

Miyasaka, K., Takata, M. and Miyasaka, K. "Flow velocity profile of the pulmonary artery measured by the continuous cardiac output monitoring catheter." *CAN J ANAESTH*, 40(2), 183- 187, 1993.

Ramsey, J. "Continuous cardiac output: Myth or reality." *CAN J ANAESTH*, 40(2), 98-102, 1993.

Woods, S., and Osguthorpe, Susan. "Cardiac output determination." *AACN Clinical Issues in Critical Care Nursing*, 4(1), 81-97, 1993.

Yeldman, M. "Continuous cardiac output by thermodilution." *International Anesthesiology Clinics*, 31(3), 127-140, 1993.

CHAPTER SEVEN

UNDERSTANDING MIXED VENOUS OXYGEN SATURATION

Mixed venous oxygen saturation (SvO_2) is a reflection of the patient's global oxygen consumption. Mixed venous oxygen saturation is obtained by either drawing venous blood gases from the distal port of the pulmonary artery (PA) catheter or inserting a continuous co-oximetry catheter with continuous monitoring capabilities.

Monitoring the SvO_2 enables the clinician to determine the relationship between oxygen supply and demand. This enables the clinician to detect subtle changes in oxygen delivery before obvious clinical changes are seen, e.g. decreased blood pressure, decreased cardiac output, or increased heart rate.

Indications for SvO2 Monitoring

SvO2 monitoring is indicated to monitor:
- Hemodynamic instability
- Multisystem organ failure
- High risk surgical patients

Methods of Obtaining Mixed Venous Oxygen Saturation

When obtaining a mixed venous oxygen sample, the nurse draws blood from the pulmonary artery. The term "mixed" refers to the mixing of blood from the superior vena cava, inferior vena cava, and coronary sinus. It is important to monitor that the catheter is in the pulmonary artery and has not migrated or pulled out. The PA waveform must be present prior to obtaining the mixed venous sample.

Mixed Venous Sample

Mixed venous sample is obtained from the pulmonary artery catheter distal port. **Table 7.1** gives the procedure for obtaining a sample.

Table 7.1. Mixed Venous Sample

♦ Using sterile technique, attach 5 cc syringe to PA distal port and withdraw 5 cc waste and discard.

♦ Attach blood gas syringe to PA distal port and slowly withdraw sample (withdrawing too quickly will cause an inadequate mix of blood to enter the syringe which may lead to inaccurate results).

♦ Flush port with pressure bag flush solution.

♦ Ensure return of PA waveform on monitor.

♦ Label specimen as mixed venous gas and send to lab on ice.

Although obtaining a mixed venous sample provides the clinician with data to assist in determining whether the patients oxygen supply is meeting the demands, it is only a measure of the patients status upon time of drawing the sample.

Continuous Mixed Venous Monitoring

Continuous mixed venous monitoring is available utilizing mixed venous pulmonary artery co-oximetry catheters. (See **Figure 7.1** on the following page.) These oximetric catheters have a special fiberoptic sensor at the tip of the catheter which analyzes the ratio of hemoglobin to oxyhemoglobin. (See **Figure 7.2**.)

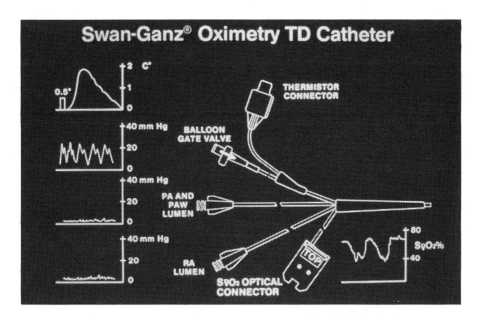

Figure 7.1. Swan-Ganz Oximetry TD Catheter. Courtesy of Baxter Healthcare Corporation, Edwards Critical-Care Division. Used with permission.

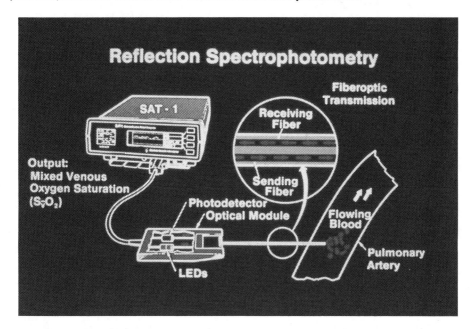

Figure 7.2. Fiberoptic tip enables continuous monitoring of SvO_2. Courtesy of Baxter Healthcare Corporation, Edwards Critical-Care Division. Used with permission.

This enables continuous SvO_2 monitoring and provides the clinician with an ongoing assessment of the patient's oxygen supply and demand.

Insertion Technique

1. Prior to insertion, the catheter is calibrated as per manufacturer's recommendations.

2. Catheter is inserted using same technique as the pulmonary artery catheter (See Chapter 3)

3. After insertion, check the manufacturer's quality index.

4. To troubleshoot the SvO_2 catheter, refer to troubleshooting pressure monitoring systems (Chapter 3) and specific manufacturer's guidelines. Difficulty with the quality index (Baxter SQI and Abbott Light Intensity Bar) is often due to one of the specific problems noted in **Table 7.2**.

Table 7.2. Problems and Troubleshooting Techniques

PROBLEM	TROUBLESHOOTING TECHNIQUE
Clot at the tip of the catheter	Attempt to withdraw clot; flush line
Catheter against the wall	Flush catheter; reposition catheter
Pulmonary artery catheter in the wrong position	Reposition catheter
Failure of the fiberoptic system (rare)	Replace catheter

Physiology

Oxygen Supply

1. Oxygen supply is the ability of the body to provide oxygen to the tissues and is influenced by the cardiac output and oxygen content.

2. Oxygen supply is also referred to as oxygen delivery. Oxygen supply or delivery is influenced by the patient's cardiac output and the content of oxygen in the arterial blood. This can be expressed as:

Delivery of Oxygen = (Cardiac Output × Oxygen Content) × 10

Note: 10 is a factor used to convert dL to L.

3. The following formula is utilized to calculate oxygen supply:

Arterial Oxygen Transport:

$DaO_2 = CO \times CaO_2 \times 10$

Normal = 1005 ml O_2/minute

Venous Oxygen Transport:

$DvO_2 = CO \times CvO_2 \times 10$

Normal = 775 ml O_2/minute

4. **Cardiac output** enables the heart to effectively pump blood out to the peripheral and coronary circulation. The normal cardiac output is 4-8 L/minute. (See Chapters 1 and 6 for further details.)

5. **Content of arterial oxygen** is derived from the amount of hemoglobin in the blood, the saturation of oxygen and a constant value of 1.38:

$$CaO_2 = Hb \times SaO_2 \times 1.38$$

Content of Arterial Oxygen = Hemoglobin $\times$ Saturation of Arterial Oxygen $\times$ 1.38

    a. **Hemoglobin** carries the oxygen. The normal hemoglobin value for males is 14-18 g/dl and females 12-16 g/dl.

    b. **Arterial saturation** is oxygen that is bound to hemoglobin. The normal arterial saturation is 95 - 100 %.

    c. 1.38 is a constant in the formula.

Oxygen Transport

Oxygen transport is the ability of oxygen to be transported to the tissues. Oxygen is carried in the blood in two forms, oxygen combined with hemoglobin (SO_2) and oxygen that is dissolved in the plasma (PO_2). The SO_2 makes up 98% of the oxygen content and the PO_2 makes up 2% of the content.

1. **PO_2** equals the partial pressure of oxygen dissolved in the plasma. The partial pressure of oxygen allows oxygen to combine with hemoglobin in the lungs and allows oxygen to be released into the tissues. This occurs by diffusion concentrations of oxygen. (See **Figure 7.3**) See **Figure 7.4** for normal partial pressure values.

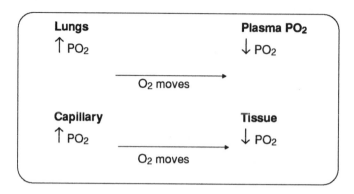

Figure 7.3. The PO_2 in the lungs and capillaries is greater than in the plasma and tissues respectively, so oxygen diffuses into the plasma and tissues.

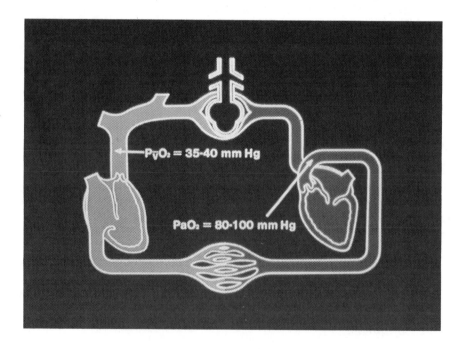

Figure 7.4. Normal partial pressures on arterial and venous side. Courtesy of Baxter Healthcare Corporation, Edwards Critical-Care Division. Used with permission.

2. **Oxygen saturation (SO₂)** is the amount of hemoglobin bound to oxygen over the total amount of hemoglobin. **Arterial blood** is normally saturated at **95-100%**. **Venous blood** is normally saturated at **60-80 %**.

3. **Oxyhemoglobin dissociation curve** tells us the relationship between the PO_2 and the SO_2.

   a. **Arterial circulation**:

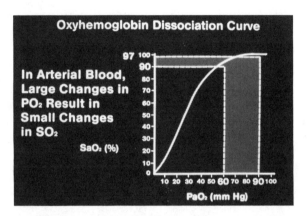

Figure 7.5. Normal arterial oxyhemoglobin dissociation curve. Courtesy of Baxter Healthcare Corporation, Edwards Critical-Care Division. Used with permission.

   • At a PaO_2 of 90, we can see that the patient's hemoglobin is saturated with 97% oxygen.

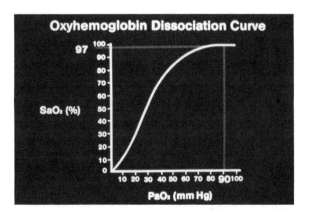

Figure 7.6. Changes in the oxyhemoglobin dissociation curve Courtesy of Baxter Healthcare Corporation, Edwards Critical-Care Division. Used with permission.

- As the PaO_2 decreases from 90 to 60, we see small changes in the SaO_2. However, there is a large change in the SaO_2 at a PaO_2 of 60 or less.

b. Venous circulation:

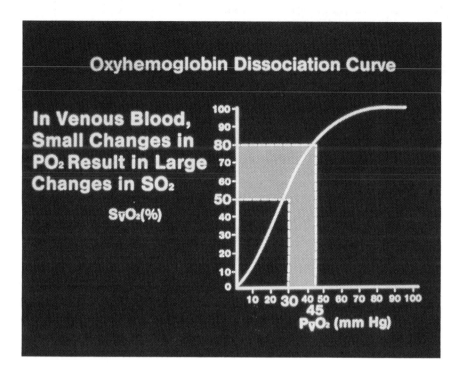

Figure 7.7. Changes in venous blood and the oxyhemoglobin dissociation curve. Courtesy of Baxter Healthcare Corporation, Edwards Critical-Care Division. Used with permission.

- As the PvO_2 (partial pressure of oxygen in the venous plasma) decreases, there is a large decrease in the patient's SvO_2. This is due to the body's ability to protect the tissues and withdraw more oxygen from the blood when needed.

c. Oxyhemoglobin affinity:

- Oxyhemoglobin affinity is the ability of oxygen to bind with hemoglobin. Increase or decreased affinity shifts the oxyhemoglobin dissociation curve to the left or right. Increased affinity means that oxygen is not released from the hemoglobin to the tissues. Decreased affinity allows oxygen to be released to the tissues. Factors affecting the affinity are stated in **Table 7.3.**

Table 7.3. Factors Which Shift the Oxyhemoglobin Curve

Shift to the Left Increased Affinity	Shift to the Right Decreased Affinity
Decreased blood temperature	Increased blood temperature
Increased pH	Decreased pH
Decreased PCO_2	Increased PCO_2
Decreased 2,3 DPG	Increased 2,3 DPG

- **Blood Oxygen Content** is the total amount of oxygen in the blood. As stated earlier, the content of oxygen is made up of the PO_2 and the SO_2. The original formula for the content of oxygen is:

Content of Oxygen $= (0.0031 \times PO_2) + (1.38 \times Hb \times SO_2)$

- Since the dissolved PO_2 comprises only two percent of the total amount of oxygen in the blood, the accepted formula to use (stated earlier) is:

$$Content\ of\ Oxygen = 1.38 \times Hb \times SO_2$$

For Arterial Content

$CaO_2 = 1.38 \times Hb \times SaO_2$

Normal $= 20.1\%$

For Venous Content

$CvO_2 = 1.38 \times Hb \times SvO_2$

Normal $= 15.5\%$

- "Common causes of inadequate transport include ventilatory failure, failure of arterial oxygenation, profound anemia, hypovolemia and myocardial dysfunction" (Mims, 1989, p. 621).

Oxygen Consumption (VO₂)

Oxygen consumption is the amount of oxygen consumed by the tissues at a cellular level. It can be defined as the amount of arterial oxygen delivered to the tissues less the amount of oxygen not used by the tissues (venous oxygen delivery). (See **Figure 7.8**)

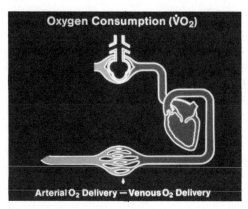

Figure 7.8. Oxygen consumption—the amount of oxygen consumed by the tissues. Courtesy of Baxter Healthcare Corporation, Edwards Critical-Care Division. Used with permission.

$$\dot{V}O_2 = \text{arterial } O_2 \text{ transport } - \text{ venous } O_2 \text{ transport}$$

$$\dot{V}O_2 = CO \text{ (cardiac output)} \times Hb \text{ (hemoglobin)} \times 13.8 \text{ (k factor) } (SaO_2{}^\dagger - SvO_2{}^\ddagger)$$

Fick equation restated

Normal 200–250 ml O_2/minute

Oxygen Balance

1. To maintain adequate oxygen balance, **Supply Must Equal Demand**.
   a. Oxygen supply:

   - As stated earlier, oxygen supply is the amount of oxygen transport to the tissues or "supplied" to them.

   b. Oxygen demand:

   - The amount of oxygen the tissues "demand" in order to meet their requirements. This is determined by the basal metabolic rate.

2. Oxygen balance is threatened by:
   a. Increased consumption (VO_2)
   b. Decreased cardiac output (CO)
   c. Decreased hemoglobin (Hb)
   d. Decreased arterial saturation (SaO_2)

†Arterial saturation
‡venous saturation

3. When oxygen balance is threatened by one of the above factors, the body attempts to compensate by increasing the cardiac output and increasing oxygen extraction (decreases SvO_2). The body is able to increase these factors by three-fold. For example:

   • In a patient with major blood loss and a drop in Hb to 6 the body will compensate for this by increasing the cardiac output and decreasing the SvO_2 (extracting more oxygen for the tissues).

$$\dot{V}O_2 = CO \times Hb \times 13.8 \times (SaO_2 - SvO_2)$$
$$= 15 \times 6 \times 13.8 \times (0.97 - 0.31)$$
$$= 819.72$$

   • Here the body extracts an increased amount of oxygen than normal to meet the requirements of the tissues. When the body is no longer able to compensate for its demands, anaerobic metabolism will occur causing the production of lactic acidosis, necrosis, and cellular death.

Mixed Venous Oxygen Saturation Monitoring

SvO_2 monitoring reflects the amount of oxygen delivered minus the amount consumed. This can be illustrated by **Figure 7.9.**

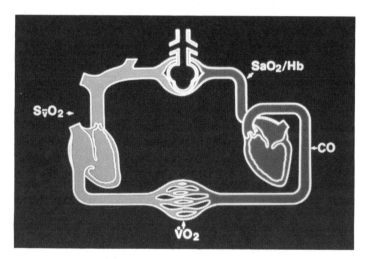

Figure 7.9. The process of oxygen supply, transport, and consumption. Courtesy of Baxter Healthcare Corporation, Edwards Critical-Care Division. Used with permission.

1. SaO_2/Hb occurs in the lungs where oxygen is bound to hemoglobin.

2. CO pumps (circulates) blood to heart and periphery.

3. $\dot{V}O_2$ oxygen consumption occurs at the cellular level.

4. SvO_2 is the amount of oxygen left in blood after tissues have consumed what is needed.

Continuous SvO_2 monitoring enables the clinician to identify early on if there are changes in the patients CO, SaO_2, Hb, and $\dot{V}O_2$. Factors that cause an increase or decrease in SvO_2 are listed in **Tables 7.4** and **7.5**.

Table 7.4. Factors That Cause a Low Svo2

Decrease in $SvO_2 < 60\%$	
Decrease in O_2 delivery	**Increase in demand**
– Low hemoglobin	– Hyperthermia
– Low oxygen saturation	– Seizures
– Low cardiac output	– Pain
– Hypovolemia	– Shivering
	– Exercise
	– Agitation
	– Burns
	– Hyperthyroidism
	– Drugs which increase metabolism

Table 7.5. Factors That Cause Increased SvO_2

Increase in $SvO_2 > 80\%$	
Increase in O_2 delivery	**Decrease in O_2 demand**
– Increased FIO_2	– Hypothermia
– Increased cardiac output	– Anesthesia
	– Neuromuscular blockade
	– Early sepsis
	– Hypothyroidism
	– Shock

When oxygen demand is greater than supply, anaerobic metabolism and lactic acidosis occurs. This causes cellular necrosis and potential destruction of tissue. The use of SvO_2 monitoring enables the clinician to make decisions to prevent the destruction of tissues and cells. It enables early recognition of the body's increased or decreased oxygen demands and provides data from which to initiate therapy. The clinician needs to evaluate the data to determine appropriate treatment for the patient.

Nursing Care and Effects on SvO₂

It is important to recognize the patient's response to various nursing activities while he or she is being monitored with an oximetric catheter. The use of the event button on the SvO_2 monitor enables the clinician to mark an event (suctioning, turning, voiding) or an activity. It is normal for the SvO_2 value to drop for 5-10 minutes, but after that time the value should return to normal. If it takes the patient longer to return to baseline, then the clinician needs to decipher the problem. **Tables 7.6** and **7.7** give potential problems which may cause changes in the SvO_2 for the clinician to troubleshoot.

Table 7.6. Troubleshooting Causes of Low SvO₂

Problem	Potential Causes
Low Hb	Anemia, bleeding
Low SaO_2	ARDS, pulmonary fibrosis, V/Q mismatch, shunting, alveolar hypoventilation
Hypovolemia	Bleeding, third spacing
Low cardiac output	Decreased preload Hypovolemia Shock
	High Preload CHF Renal failure
	High afterload Hypertensive crisis
	Low afterload

Table 7.7. Troubleshooting Causes of High SvO_2

Problem	Potential Causes
Increased FIO_2	Improved ventilation, airway patency, improved gas exchange
Increased hemoglobin	Blood transfusion
Increased cardiac output	Inotropic drugs
	Sepsis

SvO_2 monitoring can facilitate clinician determination of tolerance of therapies and routine care. When caring for the patient, the nurse performs many procedures which increase oxygen demand and consumption. By utilizing the SvO_2 monitor, the effects of nursing care on oxygen consumption can be seen. (See **Figures 7.10** to **7.12**)

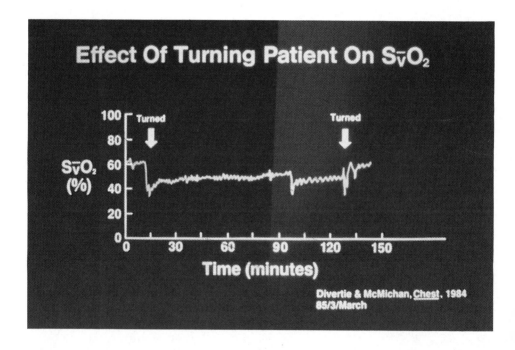

Figure 7.10. Oxygen consumption is increased upon turning patient. Courtesy of Baxter Healthcare Corporation, Edwards Critical-Care Division. Used with permission.

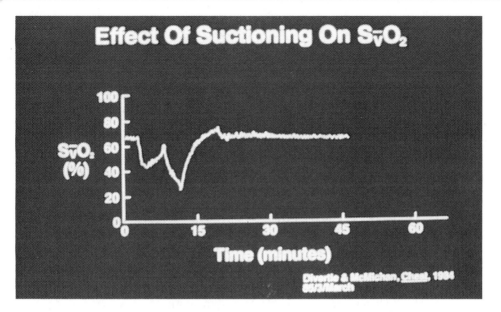

Figure 7.11. Upon suctioning there is a large decrease in patient's SvO2. Pre-oxygenation would be required for this patient to decrease the consumption. Courtesy of Baxter Healthcare Corporation, Edwards Critical-Care Division. Used with permission.

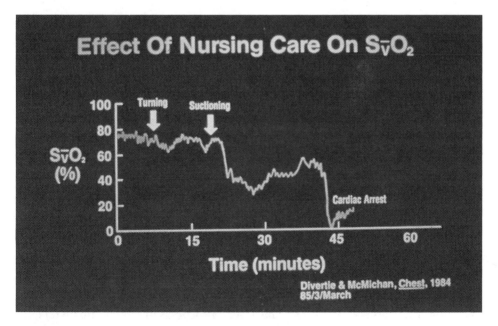

Figure 7.12. Effect of Grouping Procedures Together on the Patient's Oxygen Consumption. Courtesy of Baxter Healthcare Corporation, Edwards Critical-Care Division. Used with permission.

Selected References

Baxter Healthcare Corporation. *Understanding continuous mixed venous oxygen saturation (SvO2) monitoring with the Swan-Ganz oximetry TD system.* California: Baxter Healthcare Corporation,1991.

Clark, A., Winslow, E., Tyler, D., and White, K. "Effects of endotracheal suctioning on mixed venous oxygen saturation and heart rate in critically ill adults." *Heart and Lung,* 19(5), 552-557, 1990.

Enger, E. and Holm, K. "Perspectives on the interpretation of continuous mixed venous oxygen saturation." *Heart and Lung,*19(5), 578-580, 1990.

Gawlinski, A. and Henneman, E. "Evaluating oxygen delivery and oxygen utilization with mixed venous oxygen saturation monitoring: A case study."*Heart and Lung,* 19(5), 566-570, 1990.

Kyff, J., Vaughn, S., and Yang, S. et al. "Continuous monitoring of mixed venous oxygensaturation in patients with acute myocardial infarction." *Chest,* 95(3), 607-611, 1989.

Mims, B.C. "Physiologic rationale of SvO2 monitoring". *Critical Care Nursing* Clinics *of North America,* 1(3), 619-628, 1989.

Nierman, D., and Schechter, C. " Mixed venous O2 saturation: Measured by co-oximetry versus calculated from PvO2." *J Clin Monit,*10(1), 39-44, 1994.

Tyler, D., Winslow, E., Clark, A., and White, K. "Effects of a 1-minute back rub on mixed venous oxygen saturation and heart rate in critically ill adults." *Heart and Lung,* 19(5), 562-565, 1990.

White, K. "Using continuous SVO2 to assess oxygen supply/demand balance in the critically ill patient." *AACN Clinical Issues,* 4(1), 143-147, 1993.

White, K., Winslow, E., Clark, A., and Tyler, D. "The physiologic basis for continuous mixed venous oxygen saturation monitoring." *Heart and Lung,* 19(5), 548- 551, 1990.

Winslow, E., Clark, A., White, K., and Tyler, D. "Effects of lateral turn on mixed venous oxygen saturation and heart rate in critically ill adults." *Heart and Lung,* 19(5), 557-561, 1990.

CHAPTER EIGHT

WORKING WITH CIRCULATORY ASSIST DEVICES

Circulatory assist devices have been used to aid or support the failing heart for many years. Intra-aortic balloon pump (IABP) counterpulsation and temporary, ventricular assist support devices are being used in many institutions, especially those with heart surgery/transplant programs. This chapter includes a description of the principles and effects of intra-aortic balloon pump (IABP) counterpulsation and ventricular assist devices. Indications, contraindications, insertion site and technique, monitoring equipment, wave physiology and timing, weaning, complications and nursing care of patients with these devices will also be presented.

Intra-aortic Balloon Pump (IABP) Therapy or Counterpulsation

Principles and Effects

1. Provides temporary, mechanical circulatory assistance for the failing heart.

2. Designed to increase coronary perfusion, increase myocardial oxygen supply, decrease myocardial oxygen consumption and decrease left ventricular workload, utilizing the principle of counterpulsation.

3. Counterpulsation refers to the alternating inflation and deflation of the intra-aortic balloon during diastole and systole respectively.

4. Inflation of the balloon is timed to occur at the dicrotic notch on the aortic pressure tracing, which signifies the onset of diastole (See **Figure 8.1**).

5. Balloon inflation forces blood proximally into the coronary arteries (increased coronary perfusion pressure), the main branches of the aortic arch, and distally into the extremities.

6. Ascending aortic blood volume is therefore increased and is accompanied by a rise in diastolic pressure (diastolic augmentation). To augment something is to increase it. Since the pressure is increased during diastole by balloon inflation it is referred to as diastolic augmentation. This increases myocardial oxygen supply (See **Figure 8.2**).

7. Sufficient diastolic pressure is needed to push blood through the coronaries during diastole. Therefore a rise in diastolic pressure will help to better perfuse the coronaries or increase coronary perfusion pressure.

8. Deflation is timed to occur immediately before the aortic valve opens, or just prior to ventricular systole (See **Figure 8.3**).

9. Deflation decreases the aortic end-diastolic pressure as a result of a decrease in blood volume in the aorta.

10. As the gas is evacuated from the balloon, the pressure the left ventricle must generate to empty is reduced, hence afterload is reduced.

11. By decreasing systolic pressure, the left ventricular size, wall tension, and oxygen demands are reduced.

12. Two counterpulsation cycles are schematically depicted in **Figure 8.4.**

13. Secondary effects associated with counterpulsation include: decrease in heart rate, increase in cardiac output, decrease in systemic vascular resistance (SVR), decrease in left ventricular end-diastolic pressure or PCWP and an increase in mean arterial pressure.

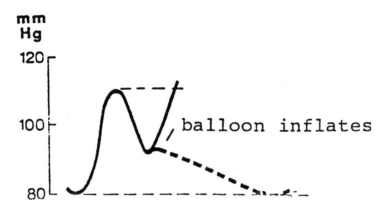

Figure 8.1. Balloon Inflation. Courtesy of Datascope Corporation, Montvale, New Jersey. Used with permission.

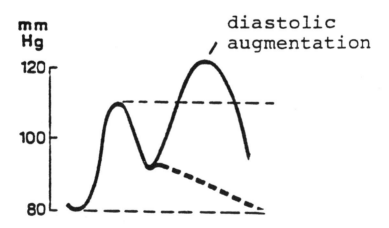

Figure 8.2. Diastolic Augmentation. Courtesy of Datascope Corporation, Montvale, New Jersey. Used with permission.

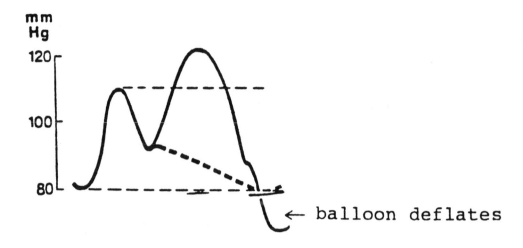

← balloon deflates

Figure 8.3. Balloon Deflation. Courtesy of Datascope Corporation, Montvale, New Jersey. Used with permission.

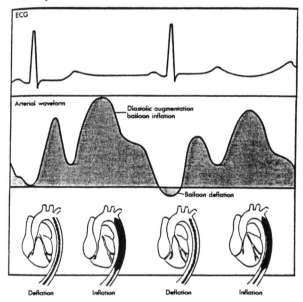

Figure 8.4. Two Counterpulsation Cycles.The balloon is inflated during diastole, thus "augmenting" diastolic pressure. Deflation occurs during isovolumetric contraction. Because balloon inflation displaces intraaortic balloon volume, aortic end-diastolic pressure is "lowered" during IAB deflation. S.J., Quaal, *Comprehensive IAB Counterpulsation,* (2nd edition) Saint-Louis: Mosby-Year Book, 1993. Used with permission of the publisher.

14. Increased mean arterial pressure will lead to improved perfusion to all organ systems. For example, as renal perfusion improves, an increase in urine output may be noted.

15. Physiological effects of IABP are summarized in **Table 8.1.**

Table 8.1. Physiological Effects of IABP

- ◆ Augmentation of diastolic pressure
- ◆ Increased coronary perfusion
- ◆ Increased mean arterial pressure
- ◆ Increased cardiac output
- ◆ Increased myocardial oxygen supply
- ◆ Decreased aortic end-diastolic pressure
- ◆ Decreased heart rate
- ◆ Decreased afterload
- ◆ Decreased systemic vascular resistance (SVR)
- ◆ Decreased left ventricular end-diastolic pressure
- ◆ Decreased myocardial oxygen demands

Indications for Use of Intra-aortic Balloon Pump (IABP)

- Cardiogenic shock or congestive heart failure.
- Unstable angina (pre or post-infarction resistant to medical therapy).
- Acute myocardial infarction with or without mechanical defects (papillary muscle rupture, ventricular septal defect, or ventricular aneurysm), or failed thrombolytic therapy.
- Ventricular dysrhythmias resistant to medications (ischemia related).
- High-risk patients undergoing interventional cardiological procedures requiring support and/or stabilization (cardiac catheterization, ventriculogram or angioplasty).
- Pre-operative assessment/stabilization of high risk patients prior to cardiac or general surgery.
- Intraoperative or post-operative support for cardiac surgery patients having difficulty being weaned from cardiopulmonary bypass, or who exhibit low cardiac output syndrome.
- Cardiomyopathy or bridge to cardiac transplantation.

Contraindications for Use of Intra-aortic Balloon Pump (IABP)

- Irreversible brain damage.
- Presence of a thoracic or abdominal aortic aneurysm with or without dissection.
- Aortic insufficiency (relative to the degree).
- Severe peripheral vascular disease.
- Chronic end-stage heart disease with no plan for cardiac transplantation.

Insertion Site and Technique

- Balloon catheter may be inserted percutaneously, by cut-down, or via transthoracic placement during cardiac surgery.
- Ideal position for the balloon is in the descending thoracic aorta, just distal to the left subclavian artery, and above the renal artery (See **Figure 8.5**).
- Placement and position should be confirmed on CXR or fluoroscopy.
- Percutaneous femoral insertion is most common. It involves threading the balloon catheter up through the femoral artery into the descending aorta (retrograde placement). Antegrade placement is accomplished via surgical approach.

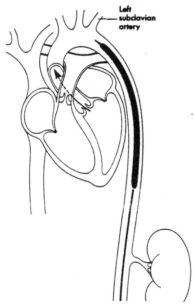

Figure 8.5. Schematic illustration of the intraaortic balloon (IAB) positioned in the descending thoracic aorta, just below the left subclavian artery but above the renal artery. S.J. Quaal. *Comprehensive IAB Counterpulsation,* **(2nd edition). Saint-Louis: Mosby-Year Book, 1993. Used by permission of the publisher.**

Monitoring Equipment

1. Hemodynamic monitoring is necessary for assessment and management of a patient requiring IABP therapy.

2. Patients will generally have a PA line, and a radial arterial line if the central lumen arterial pressure will not be used.

3. IABP consists of the balloon itself and the console that drives it. Type of balloon and console will vary depending upon manufacturer.

4. The catheter consists of a slender polyurethane balloon (usually 40 cc) mounted on a catheter with multiple pores (See **Figure 8.6**).

5. Connected to a console, it moves helium or CO_2 into and out of the balloon to inflate and deflate the balloon in accordance with the cardiac cycle (See **Figure 8.7**).

6. Console instrumentation includes a monitoring system, trigger and timing abilities, alarms and status messages.

7. Initial pump set-up consists of establishing power and selecting trigger, establishing gas pressure, setting front and rear panel controls, and establishing ECG and arterial pressure signals (Refer to specific manufacturer operator's guide). Arterial tracing must be calibrated and zeroed. (Refer to Chapter 3 for review of technique.)

8. Proper timing of balloon inflation requires an adequate arterial pressure waveform and/or an artifact clear ECG tracing. (Refer to Chapter 4 for arterial waveforms.)

9. Many manufacturers have an Auto timing mode that inflates and deflates the IAB on a beat to beat basis. The operator initially selects the inflation and deflation points; then the pump automatically adjusts for changes in heart rate.

10. Manual timing mode should be utilized for those patients who may not be optimally assisted in the Auto timing mode.

11. The "trigger" refers to the signal that the IABP system uses to identify the beginning of the cardiac cycle.

12. The R wave of the patient's ECG is most commonly used as the reference point or "trigger" for balloon inflation and deflation.

13. Other "trigger" mode settings include Pressure, Internal, Pacer V/A-V, Pacer V, Pacer A-V, and Pacer A. Refer to **Table 8.2** for further description of trigger modes.

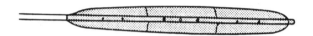

Figure 8.6. The intraaortic balloon is mounted on a vascular catheter, which contains multiple pores. Helium gas escapes through these pores and inflates the balloon. Courtesy of Datascope corporation, Montvale, New Jersey. Used with permission.

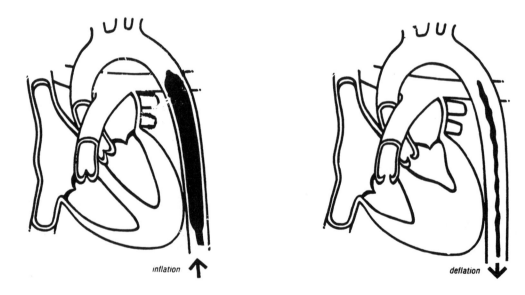

Figure 8.7. Schematic illustration of inflation of the balloon during diastole and deflation of the balloon during systole. Courtesy of Datascope Corporation, Montvale, New Jersey. Used with permission.

Table 8.2. Datascope System 97 Trigger Modes and Indications

Trigger Modes

- ECG: The R wave of the ECG is the trigger event.
- Pressure: The upslope of the arterial pressure waveform is the trigger event. With pressure trigger, balloon deflation should always be positioned before the upstroke of systole. A 15 mm Hg upstroke of the arterial pressure waveform is required to trigger the IABP.
- Internal: Used only when the patient does not have a cardiac cycle, i.e., cardiopulmonary bypass, or during cardiac arrest. The intra-aortic balloon is inflated and deflated asynchronously at a preset rate determined by the IAB frequency switch (1:1 = 120/min, 1:2 = 60/min, 1:3 = 40/min).
- Pacer V/A-V: The ventricular spike of a ventricular or an atrial-ventricular pacemaker is the trigger event provided there is a 100% paced rhythm (no demand pacing).
- Pacer V: The ventricular spike of the ventricular pacer is the trigger event. Should be used only when ECG trigger is unobtainable in the presence of a ventricular pacer and 100% paced rhythm.
- Pacer A-V: Assists 100% atrial-ventricular paced rhythms provided the A-V interval is between 80-225 msec. and the rate is less than 125 beats per minute.
- Pacer A: The R-wave of the ECG is the trigger event. Atrial pacer spikes are enhanced and rejected. Should only be used if atrial pacer spikes are interfering with R wave detection in the ECG trigger mode.

Wave Physiology and Timing of IABP

1. The arterial pressure waveform tracing is used to manually set the inflation and deflation points.

2. To evaluate the waveform effectively, the frequency should be set on 1:2 to compare the assisted and nonassisted waveforms. Freezing the waveform on the console monitor can also be helpful.

3. The dicrotic notch should be identified on the arterial tracing.

4. Inflation is usually set first, and should be set to occur 40-50 msec before the midpoint of the dicrotic notch. The dicrotic notch should disappear and a sharp V wave forms.

5. The deflation point is then set so that the balloon-assisted aortic end-diastolic pressure is as low as possible while still maintaining optimal diastolic augmentation and not interfering with the next systole (See **Figure 8.8**).

6. Optimal deflation produces a diastolic arterial pressure that is 5 to 15 mm Hg lower than the patient's unassisted end-diastolic arterial pressure, and a balloon-assisted systolic pressure that is lower than the patient's unassisted systolic pressure. **Figure 8.9** depicts the complete waveform alterations associated with inflation and deflation of the balloon, and **Figure 8.10** presents arterial waveform variations during IABP therapy.

7. Timing errors can result in sub-optimum effects of IABP therapy. **Figure 8.11** depicts common timing errors that can occur.

8. Since timing of the balloon pump is based on heart rate, any variation of heart rate may affect the performance of the balloon pump.

9. When a patient is in atrial fibrillation, the IABP should be set to inflate and deflate the majority of the patient's beats. Therapy may not be maximized due to the irregular rhythm. Atrial fibrillation trigger mode should be used if available.

10. In tachycardia, pumping every other beat may improve mean arterial pressure. The IABP frequency may be switched to 1:2.

Weaning

1. Weaning may begin when the patient's hemodynamic status stabilizes, with a gradual reduction in the amount of assistance provided by the balloon pump.

2. Optimal clinical and hemodynamic parameters include MAP greater than 70 mm Hg with little or no vasopressor support, PCWP less than 18 mm Hg, cardiac index greater than 2.0-2.5, and heart rate less than 110 beats per minute without lethal dysrhythmias.

3. Removal of the balloon should be done as soon as possible to reduce the risk of complications.

4. Weaning is accomplished by decreasing the balloon inflation frequency. It may also be combined with a reduction in the balloon volume.

5. Hemodynamic parameters must be assessed frequently during the weaning process to determine tolerance.

6. Changes in heart rate, mean arterial pressure, cardiac output, pulmonary artery pressures or mental state could indicate an intolerance to weaning.

7. Removal of the balloon that has been inserted percutaneously requires careful removal and direct manual pressure on the site for approximately 30-45 minutes (time may vary).

8. Surgery is required for removal when a balloon has been inserted via arteriotomy. The involved artery must be sutured and closed.

9. Pulses must be checked frequently following the removal of the balloon to assess the vascular status of the involved limb.

10. Vital signs and hemo dynamic parameters should be monitored every 15 minutes for the first hour after IAB removal, then every 30 minutes for the next 2 hours, and every hour thereafter as the patient's condition warrants.

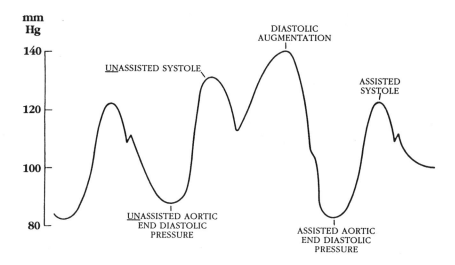

Figure 8.8. 1:2 Intra-aortic Balloon Pump Frequency. Courtesy of Datascope Corporation, Montvale, New Jersey.

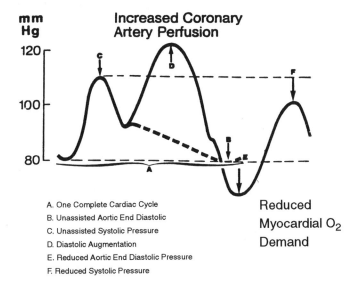

A. One Complete Cardiac Cycle
B. Unassisted Aortic End Diastolic
C. Unassisted Systolic Pressure
D. Diastolic Augmentation
E. Reduced Aortic End Diastolic Pressure
F. Reduced Systolic Pressure

Figure 8.9. Waveform alterations associated with inflation and deflation of the
balloon. Courtesy of Datascope Corporation, Montvale, New Jersey.

1:1 IABP Frequency

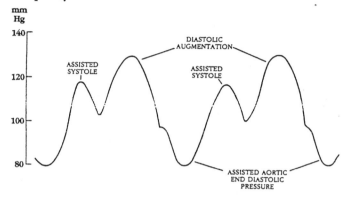

1:2 IABP Frequency

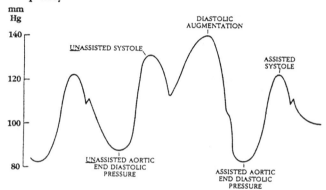

1:3 IABP Frequency

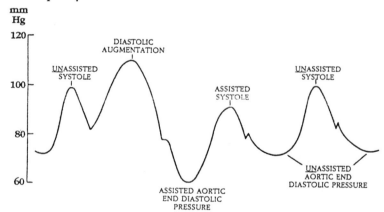

Figure 8.10. Arterial waveform variations (with varying frequency 1:1, 1:2, and 1:3) during IABP therapy. Courtesy of Datascope Corporation, Montvale, New Jersey.

Early Inflation

Inflation of the IAB prior to aortic valve closure

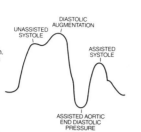

Waveform Characteristics:
- Inflation of IAB prior to dicrotic notch.
- Diastolic augmentation encroaches onto systole (may be unable to distinguish)

Physiologic Effects:
- Potential premature closure of aortic valve
- Potential increased in LVEDV and LVEDP or PCWP
- Increased left ventricular wall stress or afterload
- Aortic Regurgitation
- Increased MVO$_2$ demand

Late Inflation

Inflation of the IAB markedly after closure of the aortic valve

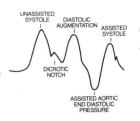

Waveform Characteristics:
- Inflation of the IAB after the dicrotic notch.
- Absence of sharp V
- Sub-optimal diastolic augmentation

Physiologic Effects:
- Sub-optimal coronary artery perfusion

Early Deflation

Premature deflation of the IAB during the diastolic phase

Waveform Characteristics:
- Deflation of IAB is seen as a sharp drop following diastolic augmentation
- Suboptimal diastolic augmentation
- Assisted aortic end diastolic pressure may be equal to or less than the unassisted aortic end diastolic pressure
- Assisted systolic pressure may rise

Physiologic Effects:
- Sub-optimal coronary perfusion
- Potential for retrograde coronary and carotid blood flow
- Angina may occur as a result of retrograde coronary blood flow
- Sub-optimal afterload reduction
- Increased MVO$_2$ demand

Late Deflation

Waveform Characteristics:
- Assisted aortic end-diastolic pressure may be equal to or greater than the unassisted aortic end diastolic pressure
- Rate of rise of assisted systole is prolonged
- Diastolic augmentation may appear widened

Physiologic Effects:
- Afterload reduction is essentially absent
- Increased MVO$_2$ consumption due to the left ventricle ejecting against a greater resistance and a prolonged isovolumetric contraction phase
- IAB may impede left ventricular ejection and increase the afterload

Figure 8.11. Timing Errors. Courtesy of Datascope Corporation, Montvale, New Jersey.

Complications

1. Complications occur frequently, with the most common being ischemia or loss of pulses in the catheterized limbs. Refer to **Table 8.3** for a list of potential complications.

Table 8.3. Potential Complications Associated with IABP Therapy

- Ischemia of the limb distal to the insertion site
- Bleeding at insertion site
- Reduced platelet count
- Infection
- Aortic or arterial damage or dissection
- Emboli from the balloon or catheter
- Balloon leak or rupture
- Pseudoaneurysm or hematoma
- Compartment syndrome after removal of IAB

2. Patients at increased risk include those with peripheral vascular disease or diabetes, older patients, and those receiving prolonged IABP therapy.

3. Other possible risk factors include obesity, shock states, smoking, and hypertension.

4. Heparin may be utilized to reduce the risk of peripheral embolic complications.

Care of Patients with IABP

1. Systematic cardiovascular assessment should be performed frequently to determine effectiveness of IABP therapy.

2. Vital signs and pulmonary artery pressures should be assessed every 15 to 60 minutes until stable. Include blood pressure (BP), heart rate, mean arterial pressure (MAP), central venous pressure (CVP), pulmonary artery pressure (PAP), and pulmonary capillary wedge pressure (PCWP).

3. Cardiac output, cardiac index, and SVR should be determined with vital signs.

4. Arterial pressure tracing should be observed frequently to assess timing of balloon, and adjustments should be made to obtain maximum hemodynamic response to IABP therapy.

5. Documentation of IABP therapy should include the unassisted and assisted systoles, diastolic augmentation, unassisted and assisted aortic end-diastolic pressures (Refer back to **Figure 8.8**).

6. Circulation to the extremities should be assessed every 15 to 60 minutes.

7. Patient is maintained on bedrest. Turn and position the patient every 2 hours, keeping the affected extremity straight. Balloon leg should not be flexed at the groin or knee. Explain to the patient the importance of keeping the affected extremity straight.

8. To reduce the risk of a pressure ulcer, utilize a specialty bed or pressure relieving mattress.

9. Head of the bed should not be elevated more than 45°.

10. Passive and active range-of-motion exercises should be instituted every 2 hours for extremities that can be mobilized.

11. Intake and output should be monitored every hour.

12. Hematologic status should be closely monitored to detect any drop in CBC or platelet count. Patient may require blood products if actively bleeding. Observe for bleeding gums, blood in urine, stool, or petechiae.

13. Anticoagulation should be administered as prescribed.

14. Area surrounding the IAB catheter insertion site should be assessed every 2 hours and as needed to note for evidence of bleeding, hematoma or infection.

Ventricular Assist Devices

Principles and Effects

1. Ventricular assist devices (VADs) provide temporary support to patients in severe heart failure who are inadequately responsive to maximal pharmacologic and IABP therapies.

2. VADs reduce the workload of the heart by decreasing preload, afterload, wall stress and myocardial oxygen consumption.

3. Temporary assist devices allow the heart to rest and recover. They are used in anticipation of recovery from ischemia or injury the myocardium has sustained.

4. The key to their success is timing and patient selection.

5. Perfusion is maintained not only to the coronaries but to all the tissues.

6. VADs can provide partial or total circulatory assistance, and are divided into three categories according to their assisting method: (1) left ventricular assist

devices (LVADs), (2) right ventricular assist devices (RVADs), and (3) combined biventricular assist devices (BVADs).

7. VADs are placed in parallel with their native ventricle, and assist with systemic or pulmonary circulation by generating 3 to 10 L/min of blood flow. Blood is pumped, not oxygenated.

8. Ventricular assist devices are of three principal designs: roller pump, pneumatic pump (air driven) and centrifugal pump.

9. Centrifugal pumps are commonly used in facilities that do not do cardiac transplantations, and are essentially pumps used for cardiopulmonary bypass. Blood flow is nonpulsatile as it is during cardiopulmonary bypass. A continuous arterial pressure is maintained for organ perfusion.

10. Long-term use is contraindicated, as VADs cannot be used for more than several days or weeks.

11. Most ventricular assist devices are still investigational, and have not been approved for use by the FDA. These include the roller pumps and pneumatic pumps. Many of these are designed for short and long-term use for patients awaiting cardiac transplant

12. The ABIOMED pump has been approved by the FDA for post cardiotomy patients. It is a pneumatic pump that provides pulsatile flow by gravity, and can supply left, right or bilateral ventricular support.

Indications for Use of Ventricular Assist Devices

- Failure to wean from cardiopulmonary bypass
- Low cardiac output syndrome following cardiac surgery
- Acute cardiogenic shock following myocardial infarction
- Bridge to cardiac transplantation
- Hemodynamic criteria may include: cardiac index less than 1.8-2.0 L/min/m^2, pulmonary capillary wedge pressure greater than 18 mm Hg, and systolic arterial pressure less than 80 mm Hg despite maximal medical therapy including IABP

Contraindications

- Poor preoperative ventricular function
- Evidence of extensive myocardial necrosis
- Uncontrollable bleeding
- Ongoing infection, sepsis, endocarditis
- Severe cerebrovascular disease or neurologic deficit
- Malignancy

Insertion Site and Technique

- In left ventricular assist, an outflow cannula is inserted into the left atrium or left ventricle to divert blood to an external assist device. An inflow cannula is then inserted into the ascending aorta in order to provide a reentry for the diverted blood.
- In right ventricular assist, the right atrial cannula or outflow cannula diverts blood from the right ventricle to the device where blood flows through the inflow cannula back to the pulmonary artery
- Following insertion of the cannulas, the chest is usually left open and covered with sterile drapes. If the patient is successfully weaned from the device, they return to the operating room for removal and closure of the sternotomy incision.

Monitoring Equipment

1. Ventricular assist devices are generally managed by perfusionists or biomedical engineers.

2. Patients are intubated, usually have a pulmonary artery catheter, arterial line, foley catheter and one or more chest tubes.

3. Hemodynamic monitoring equipment must be calibrated and zeroed as outlined in chapter 3.

Weaning

1. Successful weaning from a ventricular assist device is dependent on metabolic and functional recovery of the heart.

2. The weaning rate is approximately 50%, however only 25% of those patients are discharged alive from the hospital.

3. Once VAD insertion is completed, the patient is given maximum cardiac support for a minimum of 24 hours before any weaning is attempted.

4. To begin weaning, blood flows are temporarily turned down for 30 to 60 minutes to assess myocardial function. If function is inadequate, the flows are increased and no further weaning will be attempted for another 24 hours.

5. If weanable, a formal weaning process may be utilized. This may include a gradual reduction in flows, usually 500 ml/min every 2-4 hours until decreased to 1 to 1.5 L/min.

6. Patients are usually heparinized and the pumps are turned off for a short time before the patient returns to the operating room for removal.

Complications

Complications occur frequently, with bleeding being the most common complication. Other complications include:
- Renal failure
- Infection
- Disseminated intravascular coagulation (DIC)
- Poor cardiac output
- Thromboembolism or cerebrovascular accidents (CVA)
- Multiple organ failure
- Respiratory failure

Care of Patients with Ventricular Assist Device

1. Vital signs and pulmonary artery pressures (PAP) should be assessed every 15 to 60 minutes until stable.

2. Cardiac output, cardiac index, and SVR should be determined with vital signs.

3. Monitor VAD flow and communicate any signs and symptoms of dysfunction to perfusionists.

4. Observe for volume depletion and replace as ordered with blood or fluids.

5. Observe for signs and symptoms of cardiac tamponade.

6. Observe for bleeding from any source (chest tubes, urine, stool, GI tract).

7. Observe dressing sites for bleeding.

8. Complete daily hematologic profile: CBC, prothrombin time (PT), partial thromboplastin time (PTT), activated clotting time (ACT), fibrinogen, and fibrin split products.

9. Observe pumphead every hour for evidence of thrombi formation.

10. Administer anticoagulation therapy as ordered.

11. Assess for signs and symptoms of infection (fever, elevated white blood count (WBC), redness, swelling, and/or drainage from VAD cannulae and invasive lines).

12. Maintain aseptic technique when changing VAD lines, pumphead or dressings.

13. Patient is maintained on bedrest. Head of bed may be elevated 15°. May tilt slightly from side to side.

14. Range of motion to hands and feet only.

15. Administer antibiotics as ordered.

Selected References

Abels, L.F. *Mosby's Manual of Critical Care.* (2nd edition) Saint Louis: The C.V. Mosby Company, 1986.

Bojar, R.M. *Adult Cardiac Surgery.* Boston: Blackwell Scientific Publications, 1992.

Daily, E.K. and Schroeder, J.S. *Techniques in Bedside Hemodynamic Monitoring.* (5th edition) Saint Louis: Mosby-Year Book, Inc., 1994.

Gould, K.A. "Perspectives on intra-aortic balloon-pump timing." *Critical Care Nursing Clinics of North America,* 1 (9), 469-473, 1989.

Hudak., C.M., and Gallo, B.M. *Critical Nursing: A Holistic Approach.* Philadelphia: J.B. Lippincott Company, 1994.

Quaal, S.J. *Cardiac Mechanical Assistance Beyond Balloon Pumping.* Saint Louis: Mosby-Year Book, Inc., 1993.

Quaal, S.J. *Comprehensive Intraortic Balloon Counterpulsation.* (2nd edition) Saint Louis: Mosby-Year Book, Inc., 1993.

Shoulders-Odom, B. "Managing the challenge of IABP therapy." *Critical Care Nurse* , Vol. 11, No. (2), (60-76).

Underhill, S.L., Woods, S.L., Froelicher, E.S., and Halpenny, C.J. *Cardiac Nursing.* (2nd edition) Philadelphia: J.B. Lippincott Company, 1989.

Vaska, P.L. Biventricular Assist Devices. *Critical Care Nurse* , 11 (8),(52-60), 1991.

Wojner, A.W. "Assessing the five points of the intra-aortic balloon pump waveform." Critical Care Nurse, 6, 48-52, 1994.

CHAPTER NINE

DEMYSTIFYING PULSE OXIMETRY AND CAPNOGRAPHY

Pulse oximetry *is a noninvasive, continuous or as needed measurement of the patient's saturation of oxygen in the arterial blood (SpO_2). Pulse oximetry is available by utilizing a portable monitor which displays a digital number or as part of a modular unit that interfaces with the bedside monitoring equipment.*

Capnography *is a noninvasive, continuous measurement and waveform display of exhaled carbon dioxide (CO_2) gas that is present at the patient's airway during the entire ventilatory cycle. It is often called end-tidal CO_2, as it measures the end-tidal partial pressure of CO_2 ($PetCO_2$).*

Pulse Oximetry

Indications for Pulse Oximetry

- To provide continuous noninvasive monitoring of arterial oxygen saturation in decrease perfusion states, such as, CHF, COPD, ARDS.
- To detect immediate changes in the critically ill patient. (Limitations when PaO_2 is very high initially, e.g. PaO_2 decreases from 200 to 100, but SpO_2 will remain unchanged).
- As an adjunct to physical assessment.
- During weaning or titration of oxygen.
- For evaluating therapeutic modalities.
- As an assessment parameter in respiratory distress.
- For monitoring potential oxygen problems.

Table 9.1. Benefits of Pulse Oximetry versus ABG

Pulse Oximetry	ABG
Painless	Needle puncture
No blood loss	Blood loss
Cost-effective	Costly
Immediate results	Delayed results
Continuous monitoring	At sample monitoring
Simple technique	Skilled technique
No exposure to blood	Exposure to blood

Principles of Pulse Oximetry

1. Oxygen binds to hemoglobin in a relationship of 4:1 (oxyhemoglobin).

2. Those hemoglobins which are unable to transport oxygen are referred to as dysfunctional hemoglobins:
   - Methemoglobin
   - Carboxyhemoglobin
   - Sulfhemoglobin
   - Carboxysulfhemoglobin.

3. Pulse oximetry measures the functional hemoglobin (oxyhemoglobin), that is the relative proportions of oxygenated and deoxygenated hemoglobin.

4. Pulse oximetry measures oxyhemoglobin by **optical plethysmography** and **spectrophotometry**.

5. **Optical plethysmography** produces a graphic wave form from the changes in light absorption in a pulsatile bed. (See **Figure 9.1**)

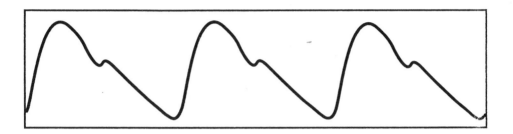

Figure 9.1. Optical plethysmography. Copyright Nellcor Incorporated, Pleasanton, California. Used with permission.

6. **Spectrophotometry** is based on the following principles:
   a. Light absorption spectra of oxyhemoglobin (O_2Hb) and reduced hemoglobin.

   b. Oxyhemoglobin absorbs more infrared light (910nm). Reduced hemoglobin absorbs more red light (660nm).

   c. A pulsatile signal generated by an arterial bed must be present (finger, nose, toe, earlobe, forehead).

   d. Pulse oximeter probe contains a light emitter and light detector located on opposite sides of the probe. The light emitter sends the signal across the pulsating vascular bed to the light sensitive detector. Since fluids and tissues do not pulsate, they do not modulate light. (**Figure 9.2**)

   e. Signal at light sensitive detector (photodetector) senses infrared absorption and transforms it into a digital display of the SpO_2 (modular units contain a wave form as well). (See **Figure 9.3-9.5**)

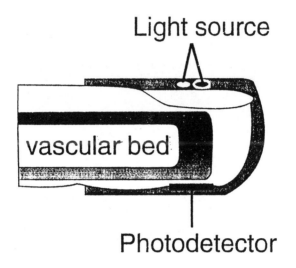

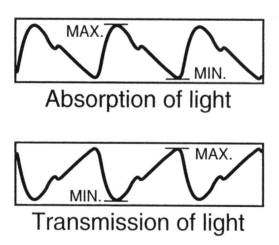

Figure 9.2. The ability of the sensor to detect pulsatile blood flow in a vascular bed. Copyright Nellcor Incorporated, Pleasanton, California. Used with permission.

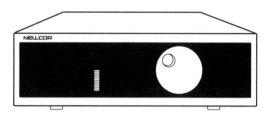

$$SpO2 = f\left(\frac{Ln\frac{max}{min}\ Red}{Ln\frac{max}{min}\ IR} \right)$$

Figure 9.3 Calculation of SpO₂ by the pulse oximeter. Copyright Nellcor Incorporated, Pleasanton, California. Used with permission.

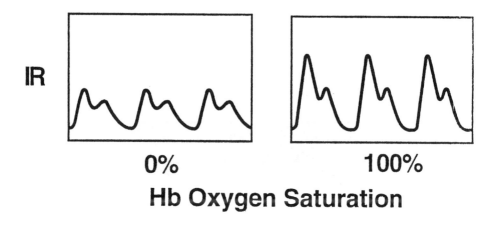

IR

0%   100%

Hb Oxygen Saturation

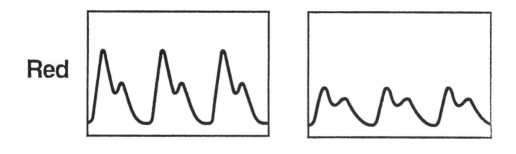

Red

Figure 9.4. The differences in light absorption of reduced hemoglobin (red light) and oxyhemoglobin (infrared light). At 0% saturation there is a greater light absorption by reduced hemoglobin, and at 100% there is a greater light absorption by oxyhemoglobin. Copyright Nellcor Incorporated, Pleasanton, California. Used with permission.

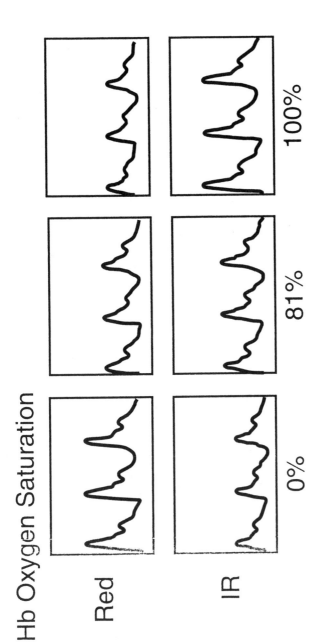

Figure 9.5. The differences in oxygen saturation of reduced hemoglobin and oxyhemoglobin. At 81% saturation you are unable to differentiate between the two. Therefore, saturations below 81% may not be accurate. Copyright Nellcor Incorporated. Pleasanton, California. Used by permission.

Relationship Between Pulse Oximetry and Oxygen Affinity

1. As the affinity of oxygen binding to hemoglobin shifts to the left or to the right on the oxyhemoglobin dissociation curve (Chapter 7), the accuracy of monitoring the patient's status via pulse oximetry is decreased.

2. In the upper portion of the oxyhemoglobin dissociation curve, large changes in the PaO_2 (partial pressure of oxygen) result in small changes in the SpO_2. This can lead to misinterpretation of the data.

Assumption of Pulse Oximetry[‡]

- All pulses are arterial
- Light passes through the pulsating beds
- Adequate hemoglobin
- No dyes present in vascular beds
- Adequate site selection
- No shift in the oxyhemoglobin dissociation curve

Equipment

- Pulse oximetry monitor or modular unit for bedside monitoring equipment
- Cable
- Probe
- Arterial vascular pulsatile bed

Choosing an Arterial Vascular Pulsatile Bed

- Site can be finger, forehead, nose, ear, or toe.
- Check for positive circulatory status and capillary refill at chosen site.
- Check for positive pulses proximal to the site.
- Avoid extremities with NIBP or arterial line in use secondary to possible interference with readings.

Selecting an Appropriate Sensor

- Wraps—use on fingers, great toe, nose.
- Clip—fingers (except thumb) and earlobe
- Headband/Forehead probe—forehead (good for those with excessive movement)

[‡]**All these criteria need to be met for values to be accurate!**

Procedure for Utilizing Pulse Oximetry

- Obtain equipment.
- Turn on monitor.
- Select site.
- Select appropriate sensor.
- Clean site with alcohol and let air dry.
- Apply sensor to patient (make sure light emitter and detector are on opposite sites of pulsatile bed).
- Connect sensor to cable and cable to monitor.
- Set alarms.
- On portable monitor, observe for pulsatile tone on machine and check accuracy by palpating patient's pulse (Note: they should be equal). Observe for digital display of SpO_2. On modular unit, note waveform of SpO_2 and digital display.

Table 9.2. Troubleshooting Pulse Oximetry Monitoring

Problem	Cause
Inaccurate SpO_2	Excessive movement
	Decreased arterial blood flow secondary to:
	Hypothermia
	Hypotension
	Vasopressor drugs
	Hypovolemia
	Decreased cardiac output
	Peripheral vascular disease
	Electrical interference
	Excessive ambient lights
	Pigmentation
	Nail polish
	Intravascular dyes
	Methemoglobin
	Carboxyhemoglobin

Loss of Pulsatile Signal	Constriction by sensor
	Reduced arterial blood flow
	Excessive ambient light
	Anemia
	Hypothermia
	Shock
Inaccurate Pulse Rate	Excessive patient movement
	Pronounced dicrotic notch on arterial waveform
	Poor quality ECG signal
	Sensor loose
	Electrical interference
	Sensor placed incorrectly

Nursing Considerations

1. Machine is calibrated by manufacturer.

2. Always keep alarms on.

3. SpO_2 does not replace an ABG measurement as it does not reflect pH, CO_2, and PO_2. Obtain initial ABG as a baseline for oxygenation to establish the relationship between PaO_2 and SaO_2 (oxyhemoglobin dissociation curve).

4. Document initial SpO_2 values and any changes in values.

5. Learn to troubleshoot SpO_2 monitor.

6. Ensure proper site and sensor selection.

7. Refer to manufacturer's guidelines before using.

Capnography

Capnography is a noninvasive, continuous measurement and waveform display of exhaled carbon dioxide (CO_2) gas that is present at the patient's airway during the entire ventilatory cycle. It is often called end-tidal CO_2 as it measures the end-tidal partial pressure of CO_2 ($PetCO_2$).

Capnometry is the measurement of exhaled carbon dioxide (CO_2) gas that is present at the patient's airway during the entire ventilatory cycle.

Capnographs are available as stand alone units or as part of modular units that interface with the bedside monitoring equipment (**Figure 9.6**).

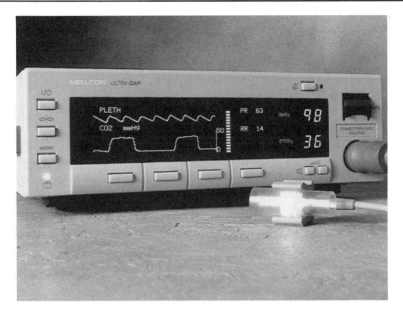

Figure 9.6. Capnograph. Photo courtesy of Nellcor Incorporated, Pleasanton, California. Used with permission.

Indications for Capnography

1. To provide continuous and noninvasive monitoring of ventilation, perfusion and carbon dioxide production in the setting of an intubated patient.

2. To verify endotracheal intubation during cardiopulmonary arrest and elective intubations.

3. To assist with weaning from the mechanical ventilator in response to changes inventilatory settings.

Physiology of Carbon Dioxide

1. **Carbon dioxide** is continually being formed in the body by intracellular metabolic processes .

2. Carbon dioxide diffuses from the cells and is transported via the venous blood to the lungs (**Table 9.3**).

Table 9.3. Transportation of Carbon Dioxide in the Blood

- ◆ Small amount in the dissolved state—7%
- ◆ In combination with hemoglobin and plasma proteins—15-25%
- ◆ In the form of bicarbonate ion—70%

3. Gas moves by diffusion from an area of greater concentration to an area of lesser concentration. Carbon dioxide gas has a diffusing capacity 20 times that of oxygen.

4. CO_2 readily diffuses across the alveolar-capillary membrane into the alveoli and is transferred to the atmosphere by ventilation. The normal range of CO_2 in the patient's exhaled gas at the end of exhalation is approximately 35-45 mm Hg. This value is the end-tidal CO_2 or $ETCO_2$ (**Figure 9.7**).

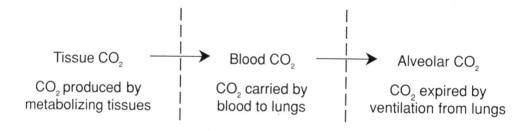

Tissue CO_2 → Blood CO_2 → Alveolar CO_2

CO_2 produced by metabolizing tissues | CO_2 carried by blood to lungs | CO_2 expired by ventilation from lungs

Figure 9.7. Carbon dioxide is eliminated through ventilation. Copyright Nellcor Incorporated, Pleasanton, California. Used with permission.

Relationship Between Arterial, Alveolar, and End-Tidal CO_2

1. Normal arterial pressure for CO_2 ($PaCO_2$) is about 40 mm Hg. The normal alveolar pressure for CO_2 ($PACO_2$) is also about 40 mm Hg. The difference between $PaCO_2$ and $PACO_2$ is approximately zero. The difference between these values rarely exceed 2 mm Hg.

2. End-tidal CO_2 is the partial pressure of CO_2 at the end of exhalation and reflects overall alveolar pressure from all functional gas exchange units.

3. When perfusion and ventilation relationships are normal, alveolar CO_2 ($PACO_2$) reflects alveolar air flow. Arterial and alveolar CO_2 are nearly equal and therefore arterial CO_2 ($PaCO_2$) reflects the state of alveolar air flow.

$PaCO_2 \cong PaCO \cong PETCO_2$

The difference between $PaCO_2$ and $PETCO_2$ is reported to be less than 6 mm Hg in normal subjects. Normally $PETCO_2$ levels are 1-5 mm Hg below $PaCO_2$. Normal ventilation/perfusion relationship must exist for this to be accurate.

Ventilation/Perfusion Mismatch $\frac{\dot{V}}{\dot{Q}}$

1. Normally there is no significant difference between $PaCO_2$ and $PACO_2$ when there are matched ventilated alveoli and perfused capillaries. In normal ventilation/perfusion, the upper lobes of the lung receive greater ventilation than perfusion and the lower lobes receive more perfusion than ventilation. The overall ventilation/perfusion ratio in the normal lung is close to 1. However, when the ventilation/perfusion ratio is abnormal, there is a mismatch and a difference exists between $PaCO_2$ and $PACO_2$ **(Figure 9.8)**.

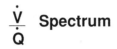

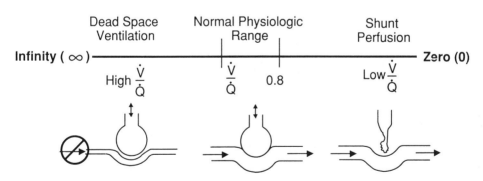

Figure 9.8. Ventilation-perfusion relationship. Copyright Nellcor Incorporated, Pleasanton, California. Used with permission.

2. **Dead Space** is the portion of inspired volume that does not reach the gas exchange unit. Anatomical dead space is comprised of the upper airway and portions of the bronchial tree (up to the terminal bronchioles) and is about 1 ml/lb of body weight. In certain lung diseases, like COPD, the alveolar dead space may become large enough to significantly affect the adequacy of gas exchange at the alveolar/capillary membrane. Lung units are being ventilated but are not perfused and therefore adequate gas exchange does not take place. In these cases, the CO_2 exhaled by the lungs ($PETCO_2$) decreases and CO_2 ($PaCO_2$) levels in the blood increases. Examples of this are: pulmonary embolus, emphysema, decreased cardiac output states, and mechanical ventilation with high airway pressures. In these cases, ventilation/perfusion ratios are high because the amount of ventilation far exceeds the amount of perfusion to these areas. The arterial to alveolar difference will be wider than normal since reduced blood flow through these areas does not allow for gas exchange to occur and exhaled CO_2 concentrations become lower than normal.

3. **Shunt Perfusion** is the perfusion of alveoli that are not adequately ventilated. This results in blood flow to the alveoli, but gas exchange does not take place. Ventilation/perfusion ratios approach zero as perfusion far exceeds ventilation. However, shunt perfusion does not contribute to abnormal widening of the $PaCO_2$ and $PACO_2$ as ventilation of normally perfused alveoli is increased to maintain a normal $PaCO_2$. Examples of shunt situations are pneumonia, mucous plugging, atelectasis, and right mainstem bronchial intubation.

Equipment for Capnography

The present status of end-tidal CO_2 monitoring in the critical care setting is comprised of an infrared light beam which passes though an expiratory gas sample (sensor) and a photodetector which measures absorption of that light by the gas. The principle is based upon the fact that CO_2 absorbs infrared light. The photodetector measures the CO_2 content and relays this information to the microprocessor in the monitor which displays the CO_2 value and wave form.

There are three types of capnographs (**Figure 9.9**). Mainstream systems mount the CO_2 sensor onto the patient's airway with the airway adapter between the endotracheal tube and the breathing circuit tubing, and measurements are made as gas flows through the airway. In the proximal-diverting systems, the measurement chamber is removed from the airway but kept close to the patient. In the sidestream system, samples of respiratory gas are withdrawn from the airway adapter positioned at the end of the tube and transported to a remote CO_2 sensor in the monitor.

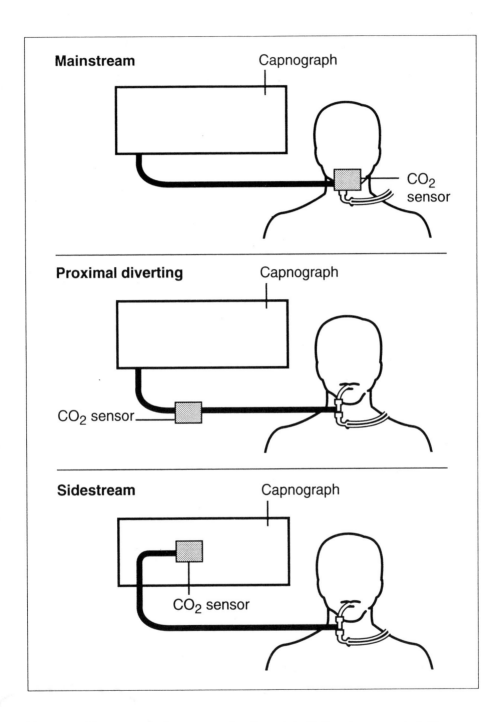

Figure 9.9. Three types of capnographs. Copyright Nellcor Incorporated, Pleasanton, California. Used with permission.

End-Tidal CO_2 Normal Waveform

Normal end-tidal CO_2 is displayed by a capnogram (**Figure 9.10**). There are four phases:

- Baseline (A-B)
- Ascending limb (B-C)
- Plateau (C-D)
- Descending limb (D-E)

As exhalation begins (point A), the sample of exhaled gas does not contain CO_2 because it will measure gas from the anatomical dead space. The steep BC segment represents the CO_2 rapidly emptying from the alveoli. The $PETCO_2$ is measured at the highest point D. The alveolar plateau is normally relatively flat as all the units have similar ventilation/perfusion relationships. The beginning of inspiration is heralded by a rapid decline (DE segment) and a decline in $PETCO_2$. Inspired gas should not contain CO_2; therefore a baseline PCO_2 of 0 mm Hg should be displayed.

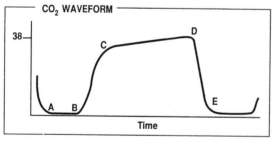

A–B:	Exhalation of CO_2 free gas from dead space.
B–C:	Combination of dead space and alveolar gas.
C–D:	Exhalation of mostly alveolar gas (alveolar plateau).
D:	"End-tidal" point—CO_2 exhalation at maximum point.
D–E:	Inhalation of CO_2 free gas.

Figure 9.10. Normal waveform. Copyright Nellcor Incorporated, Pleasanton, California. Used with permission.

Abnormal Waveforms

1. **Sudden loss of end-tidal CO_2 to zero.** Check the endotracheal tube for dislodgement; airway disconnect from the ventilator; obstructed endotracheal tube or ventilator malfunction; cardiac arrest.

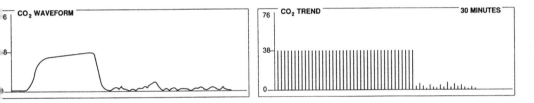

Figure 9.11. Copyright Nellcor Incorporated, Pleasanton, California. Used by permission.

2. **Gradual decrease in end-tidal CO_2.** This indicates a decrease in CO_2 production or decrease in pulmonary perfusion and/or an increase in dead space ventilation. Possible causes are blood loss, pulmonary embolus, hypotension, decreased cardiac output states. When this pattern appears on intubation, it suggests an esophageal intubation.

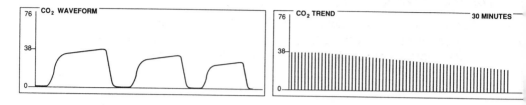

Figure 9.12. Copyright Nellcor Incorporated, Pleasanton, California. Used with permission.

3. **Sudden decrease in PETCO$_2$.** The contributing factors may be related to system leaks in airway system, disconnect from the ventilator, or of partial airway obstruction caused by secretions or malposition of endotracheal tube.

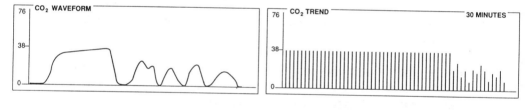

Figure 9.13. Copyright Nellcor Incorporated, Pleasanton, California. Used with permission.

4. **Sustained low PETCO$_2$.** In this situation the waveform is normal in appearance but the ETCO$_2$ value is low. This is associated with clinical conditions of dead space ventilation-emphysema, asthma, bronchitis, pneumonia, pulmonary emboli.

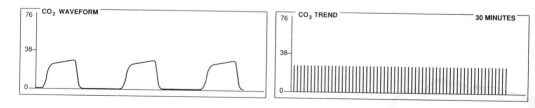

Figure 9.14. Copyright Nellcor Incorporated, Pleasanton, California. Used by permission.

5. **Gradual increase in ETCO2** is associated with increased metabolism, hyperthermia, sepsis, and hypoventilation.

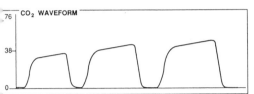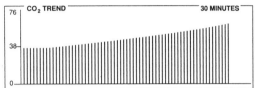

Figure 9.15. Copyright Nellcor Incorporated, Pleasanton, California. Used with permission.

6. **Sudden rise in ETCO2** suggests an increase in CO_2 delivery to the lungs. This may be associated with the release of tourniquet or bicarbonate infusion.

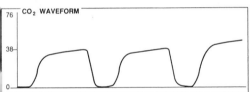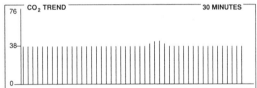

Figure 9.16.Copyright Nellcor Incorporated, Pleasanton, California. Used withpermission.

7. **Sudden rise in baseline** suggests a contaminated cell that needs cleaning.

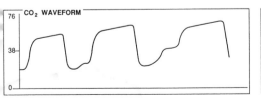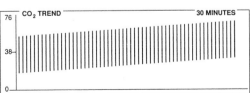

Figure 9.17. Copyright Nellcor Incorporated, Pleasanton, California. Used with permission.

Nursing Considerations

1. There is a warm-up time required for most models before full performance specifications are reached.

2. Calibration may be required by the manufacturer.

3. Turn on all alarms.

4. $ETCO_2$ does not replace ABG measurement as it does not reflect pH and O_2. Obtain initial ABG as a baseline for oxygenation to establish the relationship and gradient between the $PaCO_2$ and $PETCO_2$.

5. Document initial $ETCO_2$ values and ventilator settings.

6. Document $ETCO_2$ values along with vital signs and with changes in values and waveforms.

7. Wear gloves when handling the inline adapter.

8. Place sensor as close to endotracheal tube as possible to avoid dilution with ventilator airflow.

9. Learn to recognize normal/abnormal wave forms and correlate with causes.

10. Watch for trends in $ETCO_2$ to assess degree of deadspace.

11. Keep sensor window free of secretion, water droplets, and nebulized medications. These accumulations can produce inaccurate $ETCO_2$ results.

Selected References

Aherns, T. "The cutting edge in pulmonary critical care." *Critical Care Nurse,* Supplement, June, p 4-5, 1993.

Boggs, R. and Wooldridge-King, M. *AACN Procedure Manual For Critical Care Nursing.* (3rd edition) Philadelphia: W.B. Saunders Company, 1993.

Civetta, J., Taylor, R., and Kirby. *Critical Care.* (2nd edition) Philadelphia: J.B. Lippincott Company, 1992.

Daily, Elaine and Schroeder, John. *Techniques in Bedside Hemodynamic Monitoring.* Saint Louis: C.V. Mosby, 1989.

Daly, S. *Manual of Bedside Monitoring.* Springhouse, Pennsylvania: Springhouse Corporation, 1994.

Guyton, A.C. *Textbook of Medical Physiology.*(6th edition) Philadelphia: W.B. Saunders Company, 1991.

Nellcor Incorporated. *Arterial to Alveolar Difference for Carbon Dioxide.* Reference Note 1.

Nellcor Incorporated. *Miniaturized Mainstream Capnography* —Nellcor's ULTRA *CAP Pulse Oximeter and Capnograph.* Reference Note 4.

Nellcor Incorporated. *Advanced Concepts in Pulse Oximetry.* Hayward, California.

Osguthorpe, Susan (Editor). "Physiologic monitoring." In *AACN Clinical Issues in Critical Care Nursing.* 4 (1), 1993.

APPENDIX ONE

Vasoactive Drugs

Drug	Pre-load	After-load	Contractility	Heart rate	Blood Pressure	Cardiac output	MV O$_2$
Epinephrine	I	I	I	I	I	I	I
Isoproterenol	-	D	I	I	D	I	I
Dopamine Renal <5mcg/kg/min	D	D	-	-	-	-	-
Cardiac 5-10 mcg /kg/min	-	I	I	I	I	I	I
Vasopressor >10mcg/kg/min	I	I	I	I	I	I	I
Dobutamine	D	-/D	I	-/I	I	I	-/I
Norepinephrine	-	I	I	I	I	-/D	I
Neosynephrine	-	I	-	D	I	D	—
Amrinone	D	D	I	-/I	-/D	I	-/I
Milrinone	D	D	I	-/I	-/D	I	-/I
Nitroglycerin	D	D	-	-	D	I	-

Drug	Pre-load	After-load	Contractility	Heart rate	Blood Pressure	Cardiac output	MV O$_2$
Nitroprusside	D	D	-	D	D	I	D

Key

I = INCREASED

D = DECREASED

- = LITTLE OR NO EFFECT

APPENDIX TWO

FORMULAS AND VALUES

CHART OF FORMULAS AND VALUES

CO (cardiac output)	HR $\times$ SV	4-8 L/min
CI (cardiac index)	$\dfrac{CO}{BSA}$	2.5-4 l/min m^2
SV (stroke volume) SI (stroke index)	CO/HR SV/BSA or CI/HR	60-100 ml/beat 40-50 ml/m^2

PRELOAD
  PAS (Pulmonary artery
  systolic pressure)
		15- 28 mm Hg

PAD (Pulmonary artery diastolic pressure)		8-16 mm Hg
LVEDP (left ventricular end diastolic pressure)		8-16 mm Hg
PCWP (pulmonary capillary wedge pressure)		6-12 mm Hg
LAP (Left atrial pressure)		4-12 mm Hg
CVP (central venous pressure)		2-6 mm Hg 3-8 cm H$_2$O

AFTERLOAD
  SVR (systemic vascular
  resistance)
	$\dfrac{MAP - CVP}{CO} \times 80$	800-1200
		dynes/sec/cm^5

SVRI (systemic vascular resistance index)	$\dfrac{MAP - CVP}{CI} \times 80$	2180 ± 210 *dynes\sec\cm^5\m^2*
PVR (Pulmonary vascular resistance)	$\dfrac{\text{Mean}PAP - PCWP}{CO} \times 80$	150-250 dynes/sec/cm^5
MAP (mean arterial pressure)	$\dfrac{1\ SYSTOLE + 2\ DIASTOLE}{3}$	70-105 mmHg
LVEF (left ventricular ejection fraction)	$\dfrac{SV}{LVEDV}$	$65\% \pm 8$
SvO$_2$ (mixed venous oxygen saturation)		60-80%
SaO$_2$ (arterial oxygen saturation)		95-100%
CaO$_2$ (arterial oxygen content)	$1.38 \times Hb \times SaO_2$	20.1%

CvO2 (venous oxygen content)	$1.38 \times Hb \times SvO_2$	15.5%
DaO2 (arterial oxygen delivery)	$CO \times CaO_2 \times 10$	1005 ml O2/min
DvO2 (venous oxygen delivery)	$CO \times CvO_2 \times 10$	775 ml O2/min
DO2I (oxygen delivery system)	$CI \times CO_2 \times 10$	500-600 ml/min/m^2
VO2 (oxygen consumption)	$CO \times Hb\ 13.8(SaO_2{-}SvO_2)$	200-250 ml/min
VO2I (oxygen consumption index)	$CI \times Hb\ 13.8\ (SaO_2 - SvO_2)$	120-160 ml/min/m^2
O2ER (oxygen extraction ration)	$CaO_2 - CvO_2/CaO_2$	22-30%

The above values may vary depending on the source that is being used. When possible, the values were taken from the AACN and the Baxter Healthcare Corporation.

Index

Skidmore-Roth Publishing, Inc. Order Form
1(800) 825-3150

Qty.	Title	Price	Total
	The Nurse's Trivia Calendar	$ 9.95	
	PN/VN Review Cards, 2nd ed.	$24.95	
	The Nurse's Survival Guide, 2nd ed.	$24.95	
	The Drug Comparison Handbook, 2nd ed.	$26.95	
	Oncology/Hematology Nursing Care Plans	$27.95	
	The Skidmore-Roth Outline Series: Diabetes	$16.95	
	The Skidmore-Roth Outline Series: Geriatric Nursing	$16.95	
	RN NCLEX Review Cards, 2nd ed	$24.95	
	AIDS Nursing Care Plans	$27.95	
	AIDS Instrant Instruct	$15.95	

Tax of 8.25% applies to Texas residents only. UPS ground shipping $5 for first item, $1 each additional item.

Subtotal	
8.25% Tax	
Shipping	
TOTAL	

Name	
Company	
Address	
City	
State	Zip
Phone	

____ Check enclosed   ____ Visa   ____ MasterCard

Credit Card Number	
Card Holder Name	
Signature	Expiration Date

For fastest service call, 1-800-825-3150 or fax your order to us at (915) 877-4424. Orders are accepted by mail. Prices subject to change without notice.

Skidmore-Roth Publishing, Inc.
7730 Trade Center Avenue
El Paso, TX 79912